I0693361

After the Blue Light: One Soul's Healing Journey

A Retrospective on Surviving Through and Thriving after Emotional Trauma

Margaret-Ann Hall

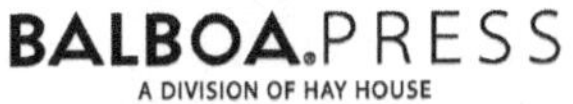

Balboa Press books may be ordered through booksellers or by contacting:

Balboa Press
A Division of Hay House
1663 Liberty Drive
Bloomington, IN 47403
www.balboapress.com
1 (877) 407-4847

Print information available on the last page.

ISBN: 978-1-9822-2809-5 (sc)
ISBN: 978-1-9822-2811-8 (hc)
ISBN: 978-1-9822-2810-1 (e)

Library of Congress Control Number: 2019906565

Balboa Press rev. date: 06/30/2020

Contents

To: Devon Alfred Yuill
Until we meet again.

Introduction

As humans we're composed of mind, body and soul (spirit). In order to lead healthy, happy, and fulfilling lives, these three aspects of our human experience must be in balance. For most of us, it's the soul that we pay the least attention to and know least about. Similar to our minds and bodies, our souls can become ill, particularly after we experience emotional trauma.

Our mainstream health and wellness systems have plenty of resources to help us treat our bodies when they're ill. As a society, we're finally beginning to recognize mental illness as a real disease, and resources to treat the mind are becoming more acceptable and available all the time. However, treatments for the soul are still relatively unknown and not readily available in most areas.

To help you understand how to heal your soul after emotional trauma, you must first understand what your soul is and the crucial role it plays in your life. This book explains how I learned about my soul, how I determined it was ill, how I healed it, how I picked up the pieces of my life, and how I found happiness and fulfillment.

I'm an unlikely candidate to have written a book that focuses on the soul. I have a bachelor of science degree. I majored in computer science, and I have thirty-two years of experience in the information technology industry. I've been a consultant for twenty of those years and have been self-employed for the last fifteen years. Although I worked and lived in the United States for a short time, I've spent the majority of my career working in eastern Canada.

I've worked hard and I've had good success in my professional life, but finding success in my personal life remained elusive for many years. As a child, I was verbally, physically, and emotionally abused at the hands of my mother. In my mid-thirties, I experienced a painful divorce when my only child (a daughter) was three years old. For the most part, I've provided for and raised her by myself. She is now twenty-two years old and attends a small university in eastern Canada.

Despite my less-than-ideal upbringing, I've beaten the odds. I consider myself to be a survivor. That doesn't mean I didn't struggle, and I most certainly didn't make it here alone. I had the support of some incredible people (my earth angels) and professional counseling, and I made it my mission to read every self-help book I could get my hands on. In addition, my life has also been influenced by some very profound, serendipitous, and spiritual experiences.

Over time, without realizing it, I took everything I learned from those people, experiences, and books and developed a belief system that has helped me break the cycle of abuse and become a successful parent and business owner. Living by the concepts I describe in this book, I found the strength and courage to make some incredibly tough choices and change my life for the better.

I've also leveraged these concepts, in conjunction with the law of attraction, to influence and manifest my own destiny. Instead of getting caught up in the emotions, I'm now able to stand back and look at my life, during those times when it's uncontrollably unraveling in front of me, and have comfort that things will eventually work out, in ways that I could never have imagined.

Although the concepts I describe in this book may be new to you, they're not new concepts. In fact, they've been around for centuries. They just haven't become part of mainstream thinking yet. I believe that these concepts are bubbling closer and closer to the surface and we're about to reach a tipping point. For that reason, I've placed quotes from famous (and not so famous) people, at key points throughout this book to reinforce the fact that I'm not alone in my thinking. Others have used these concepts to improve the quality of their lives as well.

By paying attention to and taking care of your soul, you have the power to start improving the quality of your life the minute you finish reading this book, but first, you have to have an open mind. If you find yourself resisting some of the content in this book (perhaps feeling conflict with your religious beliefs or your educational background or both), remember that I experienced that same resistance at periods throughout my life. As you progress through this book, I encourage you to stretch the boundaries of your mind and your belief systems and keep reading.

I've read many self-help books, and not all the content resonated with me. Despite that, I found nuggets of wisdom in each of them. If you're looking to improve the quality of your life, then the messages and concepts I convey in this book can help you. If you find yourself resisting, try to hang in there and look for your nugget.

Section 1

Connecting and Communicating with Your Soul

So often we look to external sources to validate and guide us through this journey called life. This is unfortunate because we have the one expert, our very own life coaches, our souls, along with us, as our constant companions. The trick is to learn to tune in and listen to the endless guidance (aka intuition) that our souls provide.

Unfortunately, it's not a perfect system, and it's not always easy to tune in. Life comes with many obstacles that hinder us from listening to our souls. These obstacles present themselves to us in many forms:

- conflict with conventional mainstream wisdom
- conflict with our education in the sciences
- conflict with religious beliefs
- fear and doubt

To add to the complexity, listening and acting on guidance from our souls may mean taking an emotional or financial risk, going against the advice/wishes of loved ones and/or being judged by our peers.

If our souls are available to offer guidance, where does that guidance come from? What is our soul?

What Are Our Souls?

Our souls are our true selves and our true essences. They're who we really are. When we think of the triumvirate of the mind, body and soul, the mind and body are only temporary. The soul is eternal. In our truest state, our souls are simply a form of energy. Comprised of pure love, its primary purpose is to guide and encourage us to lead fulfilling lives and to live our lives authentically.

Even with my Christian upbringing, I doubted the existence of an eternal soul. I now emphatically know the soul is eternal and exists beyond the boundary of our body and even this planet earth, because of two profound personal experiences. Before I recount them, it's probably worth noting, that I don't indulge in hallucinogenic drugs. The first experience happened in early 2004.

While I was sleeping in my bed, I was pulled from my body and taken on a journey through an ethereal blue tunnel of light. As I traveled along this blue tunnel of light, I experienced weightlessness and total freedom from my physical body. Tiny white lights whizzed by me as I followed the twists and turns and accelerated through the tunnel. I've never traveled at the speed of light, but I believe I did that night. As I progressed through the tunnel, a feeling of pure ecstasy came over me. I was bathed in bliss, and as I felt these incredible sensations, I had this overwhelming sense of knowing that I was going "Home." And I couldn't wait to get there.

I'm not sure if I actually reached Home that night. If I did, I have no memory of it. What I do remember clearly are the feelings I had as I returned to my body. I felt myself slowly hovering and lowering over my body. Then the weightlessness quickly dissipated as I started to feel the weight of my arms and legs again. This was when my physical body woke up. My eyes opened at that time, and I became aware of the tingling sensations throughout my entire body. The feelings of pure love and bliss remained with me for a while but eventually disappeared as I laid there and wondered, *What the hell just happened to me?*

Although the memory of that first experience stayed with me for a while, I discounted it, convincing myself I'd just imagined it, and eventually mainstream thinking led me to push it out of my head entirely. It wasn't until many years later, during my second encounter with Home, that I finally decided my first experience was real. During my second experience, I didn't travel Home. Instead, I was offered a "glimpse."

In my mind's eye, I saw what my soul really looks like. Comprised of white light, it's a crystal-like structure that's constantly pulsating and dynamically changing shape. Several light beams emanating from the bottom of the crystal gradually transition from white to a light blue as they integrate with a base of pulsating blue light. As I stared at it, I instinctively knew it was the "real" me.

I could see other crystals (i.e., other souls) adjacent to me and attached to the base of blue light as well. Together, we form one mind, that I typically refer to as the "collective conscience." Although I don't fully understand it, our souls don't experience time there. We simply exist in states of pure love.

While I stared at the crystal, I recalled a few pages I'd read in a book I'd pulled from a library shelf while looking for a distraction from my studies in university. I didn't read the book for long, as the concepts made no sense to me until the moment I saw my soul, and then it all clicked.

The book explained that, at the time of our conception here on earth, a piece of our soul joins with our human bodies and minds. It's a symbiotic relationship in that none of the three can exist here on earth without the others. While our souls are inhabiting our bodies here on earth, they're still connected to the blue light of Home. Until the day our physical bodies expire, we're *always* connected. It's that connection that gives us the potential and power to shape our own lives.

I'm not sure where Home is. I don't claim to have all the answers, as I've chosen to only convey in this book what has been shown and communicated to me. What I refer to as *Home* has sometimes been called *the Source*, and some might even consider it to be *heaven*. For reasons which I'll explain later, I don't think in or use religious terms anymore. I tend to think that all aspects of our spiritual world (Home) and our physical world (Earth, our solar system, and the galaxy) come together to form the universe, and I believe the universe is sentient.

> We are not human beings in search of a spiritual experience. We are spiritual beings immersed in a human experience.
>
> —Wayne Dyer

I recognize this book may be reading like something from a bad science fiction novel. That's not a mistake. There are many people having similar experiences and receiving similar messages from Home. Some are ignoring those messages (as I did for a long time), while others are choosing (or being guided) to communicate the messages in different ways, through different mediums (e.g., books, movies, blogs, podcasts).

Anyone who has specialized in business communications will tell you that the best way to get a message understood is to distribute it often, in diverse ways (because we all process and absorb information differently), and to as many people as possible. Our souls are constantly trying to communicate with us about Home and our purposes here on earth. For those of us who eventually listen, it's clear that our souls not only want us to listen to the guidance but also want us to communicate the role the universe plays in helping us receive and act on that guidance.

Prior to writing this book, I had only shared these experiences with a handful of "safe" family, friends, and practitioners. This was because I feared being judged and labeled as insane or eccentric. (I'm neither.) In those rare occasions when I remembered my trip into the blue light, the memory of the feelings of love and bliss drove me to ponder: "If that's what Home really feels like, then why would my soul want to come here?"

Why Do We Come Here?

This is the ultimate existential question, and (once again) I don't claim to know the complete answer, but I will share what has been revealed to me.

We come here to experience life on a different level. Our souls want to feel what it's like to breathe air and to experience what it's like to taste, touch, feel (other emotions besides love), hear, and see. We also come here to separate from the collective conscience and to develop and distinguish ourselves as individual souls.

Even with the vivid memories of my trip into the blue light, for many years I downplayed the experience because I could not reconcile it against my education in the sciences. I just couldn't understand how, if these two different worlds existed, it was possible to communicate between here and there (earth and Home). I recognize that this may not bother most people, but because I understand the science behind telecommunications (i.e., communication needs a medium—it can't happen in a vacuum), I just couldn't rely on blind faith. I needed to understand, in scientific terms, how this could happen.

This caused me to abandon my spiritual inquisitiveness and growth throughout periods in my life. However, for one reason or another (typically during or after a traumatic event or trying times), I kept being drawn back to continue my spiritual development. Oddly enough, it was my knowledge of the sciences (particularly physics) that helped to reconcile the conflict within and allowed me to finally commit to my spiritual growth and beliefs.

If the only way we can successfully navigate our lives and find fulfillment is to connect and communicate with Home, how is it possible to communicate between here and there?

Everything Is Energy—Part 1

If you study physics, you know that energy exists in everything in the universe. Science has proven that every object (even human DNA) has a **resonant** frequency—the natural frequency at which something vibrates.

As any two objects approach one another, their energy fields begin to interact. If both objects are vibrating at the same frequency, they can interact and sometimes even communicate (especially if both objects are sentient) with one another. If they're not at the same frequency, they coexist in the same space, but there is no potential for communication between the two.

One of the best examples to demonstrate this phenomenon is a singer shattering a piece of glass. In their natural states, a human and a piece of glass don't share the same resonate frequency. Placed side by side, they can coexist, but they cannot communicate with one another. However, if the human begins to sing and creates sound waves that match the resonate frequency of the glass, the glass will begin to vibrate (the point at which communication could occur) and may even shatter.

Thankfully, our souls aren't as rigid as glass. When we're here on earth and interacting with the energy from Home, we align with one another to create a conduit through which messages (i.e., guidance) can pass without harming either side.

This is a very rudimentary science lesson, and I apologize to those who've written entire books on the subject. Please know my intent isn't to discount their efforts or their field in any way. My intent is to explain the concepts with brevity and in a way that (I'm hoping) anyone can understand.

Although we cannot see or touch the energy of Home around us, it's constantly flowing around and through us. If you're someone who's already connected and receiving messages, you'll understand what it's like to communicate with Home. For those who are new to these concepts, I can tell you that you may have already unknowingly communicated with Home. It's that moment when your hair stands on end, your body tingles, and you get goose bumps because something you experienced just completely resonated with and touched your soul.

Pay attention and celebrate those moments in your life. They're confirmation that your conduit is open and you're able to receive messages. Tune in and try to seek out more of those moments. That may help you discover your aha moment, or that point when you start believing. Because believing, is the foundation for establishing connection.

> The energy of the mind is the essence of life.
>
> —Aristotle

I went through much of my life not connecting with my soul, but as I became more aware of my soul, I started to wonder: Why is it so important to listen? What's been the impact of not listening?

The Importance of Connecting and Making the Right Choices

In an effort to distinguish ourselves from the collective conscience, our souls come here with unique plans to develop and grow as individuals. This implies that there is a predetermined path, a straight line from our births to our deaths. But it's not quite like that, because the universe provides us with unlimited choices and the power to make the decisions to carve our own paths and take our lives in any direction we choose.

Very simply put, the way we navigate our paths from life to death is very similar to getting in our cars and driving to destinations. Typically, we have any number of routes to get us there, and some routes can be more enjoyable than others. Regardless of how we finally reach our destinations, the routes we choose can have direct impacts on the quality of the journeys. Perhaps we chose a route with an unexpected detour that brought us to a beautiful place we wouldn't otherwise have seen or a person we would never have met. Conversely, a detour could cause us to miss experiences that would have enhanced our journey.

Ultimately, our paths in life are determined and defined by our choices. It's not so much that we can make wrong choices. Sometimes there just may be a better choice. That's why staying connected is so important, because it helps us receive the guidance to make the best choices to live our lives authentically and be the best versions of ourselves. When we're living authentically, life is satisfying, rewarding, and we feel "fulfilled."

Some people have been lucky to lead fulfilling lives and may have never been consciously connected. That's because the choices that made them happy also fed their souls and led to fulfillment. This isn't to say that if we choose not to be connected and have strayed from our path, we can't feel some sense of happiness. It's been my experience that we can feel happy but at the same time feel unfulfilled.

The difference between the two emotions is that feeling happy is a state that's associated with the mind, while feeling fulfilled is a state associated with the soul. To lead a balanced life, between the mind, body and soul, both feelings need to be present.

Time and time again, we witness people who've achieved great wealth and success but who appear to be miserable. We only need look to the current string of celebrity suicides to recognize this is a common occurrence. It's likely that their successes may not have brought them fulfillment because they didn't earn those successes by being authentic and true to themselves. This doesn't mean they earned their success illegally; it just means they likely weren't connected and paying attention to their souls while they were achieving their successes.

In not paying attention to their souls, they shifted the balance between happiness and fulfillment and inadvertently created an empty space. It's that empty space that generates feelings of unfulfillment. Many people refer to that empty space as "the void."

I have observed that some people are okay experiencing the void, while others are very uncomfortable with it. Those who are uncomfortable try to mask or fill the void with other things. The list of things is long, but the more common ways to fill the void is turning to drugs (both legal and illegal), alcohol, food (i.e., becoming emotional eaters), or other people (i.e., changing partners or having affairs). Since most people don't understand the origins of the void, it can exasperate them to the point where the feelings of unfulfillment begin to shift and affect their feelings of happiness; sometimes leading to depression.

At the age of thirty-five, I had everything I'd ever wanted in my life. I was married, and I had a beautiful daughter (she was a toddler at the time), a gorgeous four-bedroom home in the suburbs, and a quaint little cottage on a lake. I was happy, but there was something missing. Looking back (I didn't know it at the time), it was because I wasn't connected to my soul, and despite achieving everything I wanted, I was miserable. I was feeling the void.

My family doctor diagnosed me with depression, prescribed antidepressants, and started me off with a small dosage. I felt lighter and happier for a while, but eventually, the feelings of unfulfillment returned. I went back to my doctor, and she increased the dosage. My mental state improved for a short time, but eventually, I started feeling the void again.

This cycle continued until I reached the conclusion that antidepressants weren't the answer for me. At this point, exasperation was taking over, and I couldn't understand what was wrong with me. My doctor recommended professional counseling. It didn't take long for my counselor to point out that much of my unhappiness was likely caused by the unhealthy relationship I'd created with my husband. Unhealthy marriages are all too common, for people who were raised in less than ideal circumstances.

It's a shame I wasn't capable of coming to that conclusion on my own. Through counseling I've come to realize that the dynamics of my relationship with my mother, skewed my perception of what was normal. I also learned that being an abused child left me with deep-rooted feelings of vulnerability and insecurities as an adult. Many people use aggression to compensate for their insecurities. Instead of becoming aggressive myself, to compensate for my insecurities, I sought out overly aggressive males for my intimate relationships. In a way, I mistook their aggression for confidence.

After I sought counseling, not only was I feeling the void, I realized (in some ways) I was reliving my dysfunctional childhood. In retrospect, I had strayed from my best path in life. That's when we can look for something else to fill the void or make the choice that will start us back on a better path. These are the defining moments in our lives.

The choice I wanted to make at that time (efforts to repair the relationship were unsuccessful) was to dissolve my marriage. But divorce comes with such a social stigma. I just didn't have the confidence, nor the courage, to take that step in my life. That's the problem with making some of these choices to put us on better paths in life—they typically require us to go against the grain of mainstream thinking or our religious beliefs and put us in a place to be judged by our peers, friends, and family.

In addition, these tough choices usually force us to look inward, develop self-awareness, stop seeing ourselves as victims and blaming others for the state of our lives, and take responsibility for our actions, our choices, and ultimately our lives. This is extremely difficult if (like me at the time) we're very insecure, worry what others think, and let others make our choices for us. As long as we let others influence or decide our path in life (or are afraid to make the tough choices), we will likely feel the void.

If we're feeling that void, chances are there's a better choice (we may already know what it is) we're not making. That's why it's so important to be connected to Home, because the guidance we receive gives us the courage to make those tough choices and get our lives on better paths. Staying connected can also provide us with encouragement (to keep us moving forward during those difficult times) and can even celebrate when we're finally back on better paths. Connect with your soul (and Home). Tune in and listen. You'll be guided to safer ground.

How do we recognize guidance from Home?

Recognizing Guidance

Although the concept of guidance from Home hasn't fully penetrated mainstream thinking, there's awareness of something similar, and it's referred to as *intuition*. Regardless of the terminology, guidance comes to us in many forms, and how people receive guidance is unique to each individual. It's not enough just to recognize guidance, as you may also have to interpret it because the meaning isn't always clear. It's not the intent of this book to provide in-depth instruction on recognizing and interpreting guidance—many books have already been written on the subject. Instead, I will explain how I typically receive guidance and some of my more memorable experiences.

Guidance typically comes to me as words or short phrases that I hear in my mind. On rare occasions, I'll see images through my mind's eye and receive messages through deceased loved ones. Sometimes I'll just experience a very strong sense of knowingness. I usually don't have a problem recognizing guidance, but interpreting guidance didn't come naturally to me. Through much practice and trial and error, I've become pretty good at interpreting the messages.

I find the best time to receive guidance is early in the morning when I first wake up. It's during those times that my mind is fresh and quiet and the noise of my day has not yet created interference or distractions. I'll pose a question and listen for an answer. I try to avoid questions that would solicit yes or no responses. This method prevents my bias from inadvertently influencing the response to the question. When a response seems to be "out of the blue," and not related to anything I was thinking at the time, I know for sure it's guidance. I also use this same technique during or after meditation.

The last paragraph describes the most common method I use when I'm actively seeking guidance. However, there have been times when I've received guidance and didn't explicitly ask for it. One such case came to me from an unlikely source before I understood what it meant to be connected and when I needed it most.

After I realized my marriage was unhealthy, I wanted to end things, but I didn't have the courage to make the tough decision, and I also believed I couldn't make it on my own. I was at the point where being stuck and not making a decision felt better and less daunting than dissolving the marriage. It was around that same time that my mother died very suddenly. Although I didn't have a great relationship with my mother, I was deeply affected by her death. Along with feeling unfulfilled, I was also feeling grief, and then I fell into despair. I became paralyzed and frozen.

Then about six weeks after my mother passed, she came to me in the middle of the night. It wasn't a dream, because it felt so real. It was a very short vision that only lasted between fifteen to twenty seconds. Although my physical body was asleep, I felt awake. I tried to speak, but she interrupted me. She told me to leave the marriage, as it would never be healthy for me and my daughter. Then she put her arms around me and hugged me and quickly disappeared. I could actually feel that hug. I can still feel it to this day. I believe that vision was my mother's way of making up for her poor parenting skills here on earth.

As someone who felt unloved much of my childhood, that vision was a gift, and it gave me the strength to start divorce proceedings. Each time fear, doubt, and insecurities crept in, I used the vivid memory of my mother's visit, the feeling of that hug and her advice, to keep moving forward.

> One of the most courageous decisions you will ever
> make is to finally let go of what is hurting your heart
> and soul.
>
> —Brigitte Nicole

This is an example of guidance from a departed loved one. Since all souls are part of the collective conscience, your departed loved ones have access to use your connection to Home and can use it to communicate with you.

There are times when there has been no verbal communication and the guidance I receive just comes through as a very strong sense of knowingness. In other words, things just feel right.

In the months leading up to the end of my marriage, I began envisioning myself and my daughter living in a semidetached home on a quiet cul-de-sac with plenty of children for her to go outside and play with. On the day we'd gone looking for our new home, I had viewed several semidetached houses and found a brand-new one on a quiet cul-de-sac. Although it was a little above my price range, I made up my mind that this would be our new home.

However, my real estate agent said, "I have one more house to show you." Thank goodness he was more about finding me a good home instead of making money. Because the next house we looked at was also on a quiet cul-de-sac, but it was a little cheaper, a little older, and a little smaller. I still can't describe the feeling when I walked in to the front door. I just *knew* it was my home.

Once I made the decision to buy the cheaper home, things just fell into place. Eventually, I realized I had less money than expected and I was short $1,500 for the down payment. Coincidentally, my bank was offering a $1500 rebate (an offer that I couldn't have taken advantage of with the first home I picked, because it was new construction).

We lived in that home for fourteen years. We quickly made friends, who eventually became like family. I could never have imagined the support I'd have received as a single mom. There were plenty of kids and my daughter spent her days playing with them, while we parents sat on the sidelines refereeing. Now, as young adults, they're more like siblings than friends.

In the years since, I have often thought about what my life would have been like if we had purchased the newer home. Both houses were in the same neighborhood, so I may have met my neighbors in some other way. However, I believe the quality and depth of the relationships were forged because we spent so much time together, and that just wouldn't have happened if we hadn't lived so close to one another. I believe it would have been one of those instances where I was close to the right path but not quite there. I'm sure my life would have been good, but not as good as it was.

These experiences have all been instances where the communication I received from Home was clear and easy to interpret. However, I regularly receive guidance that's more challenging to interpret, in the form of random coincidences. This type of guidance requires you to pay close attention because what originally appears to be unrelated events can eventually become linked and very meaningful.

Random coincidences can be something as simple as when you think of a person and they call you. Or money showing up (like the $1,500 rebate, when I purchased my home) just when you need it. I can usually tell it's guidance because I feel what I can only describe as a little ripple in the back of my mind. It's not something physical; it's just a slight change in my mental state. Just enough to poke me and say, *Pay attention!* Chances are that if you're asking yourself if this coincidence means something, it does! Stop what you're doing and take notice of everything that's happening around you.

What I've learned about interpretation of random coincidences is that they can serve a couple of purposes. At times, they just seem to be confirmations and celebrations that your life is on the right path. Other times, they can act like beacons to help nudge you down a particular path when you're making difficult life choices.

Sometimes, I can eventually tie what initially appear to be random coincidences together into a string of meaningful coincidences. They can appear clustered together over a short period, or they can be stretched out over a longer interval. This is called "synchronicity" and is the reason I always journal my coincidences. This allows me to analyze my coincidences over time so I can notice patterns and determine if there is a larger message. Synchronicity is guidance that points you toward a certain path or choice.

After the divorce and after the move into the new home, I focused on providing a healthy environment to raise my daughter. I was much happier because I was no longer in an unhealthy relationship, but I was still feeling the void. This led me to spend a lot of time reading self-help books and deepening my spiritual beliefs. Looking back now, I was starting to become aware of the reasons for the void. I was beginning to understand about the connection to Home. I wanted to learn to connect with my soul, but I wasn't having a lot of success. I was starting to wonder if my connection to Home was impaired and if my soul might be sick.

I had a very difficult time finding local resources to help me, and it was at this time that I noticed the lack of resources in our mainstream health and wellness systems that deal with the soul. We have practitioners to help us heal our bodies and minds, but there are no mainstream, Western-world resources that help us heal the soul.

I did my research on the web and determined that Sedona, Arizona, was home to many spiritual retreats for those looking to cradle, heal, and communicate with their souls. It's believed to be the heart center of the earth. The energy in Sedona vibrates at some of the highest levels here on earth. Having been there a number of times, it now feels like another home, but taking my first trip there (by myself) was very intimidating.

My only sibling (a sister) lives in Phoenix, so taking a trip to Arizona (by myself) wasn't a stretch for me, but driving north of Phoenix and out into the desert alone was. I didn't know anyone there. I'd be alone in a strange place, and the price tag of the retreat was hefty. I was afraid I'd be throwing my money away.

However, as I started down the path of evaluating different retreats, I noticed some interesting things started to happen. As I was on the phone talking to one of the retreat owners, I looked out my office window and noticed an eagle flying overhead. I thought that was rather odd, as I'd never seen an eagle in the city before. By this time, I'd read several books on synchronicity and coincidences. I took the appearance of an eagle in that moment as a huge sign (i.e., guidance). I made that leap of faith, and I booked the retreat.

Then, as I went to book airline tickets on the web, I noticed the banner on the home page for the airline had an eagle on it. As I progressed through the web pages, I used the eagle in the banner on top of the page as encouragement to keep moving forward. Just like a path of bread crumbs, I followed the eagles on the web-page banner to the point where I purchased the ticket. It was exciting and terrifying at the same time.

Months later as I drove into Sedona for the first time, I prayed I'd see an eagle as confirmation that I had done the right thing. To my shock and amazement, there were statues of eagles everywhere. Unbeknownst to me, eagles are a big part of the culture in Sedona.

During that trip I met with several practitioners who helped me connect with and heal my soul. For the first time in my life, I felt like my mind, body and soul were balanced. It was also during that trip to Sedona that I first started dabbling with the law of attraction and when I put it out to the universe that I wanted to make more money, work less, and have more flexible working hours.

Over the course of the following year, a number of other random coincidences and nudges happened. I journaled them, linked them (i.e., synchronicity), and did my best to follow and interpret the signs. Eventually, I was offered a one-year contract, and I quit my full-time job and started my own consulting business. As a single mom, this was a huge risk for me to take. In those early days, I was terrified, especially on the first day of my new contract with my new client. However, I was relieved, amused, and grateful, when I was assigned my temporary password. It was "theeaglehaslanded." I took it as complete confirmation and a celebration that I had made the right choice and was on the right path.

I've worked steadily for the past fifteen years (a sure sign I was on the right path), and I've never looked back. I found the flexibility I required (my daughter eventually became a competitive swimmer, and I had to leave work most days at three forty-five to get her to practice). I found clients who supported me. In turn, I worked hard to help them be successful in their careers (which was rewarding for both of us). I was able to take six-to-eight weeks off every year (as opposed to four weeks), and I had more disposable income. Every intention I set in Sedona had become a reality.

I took a couple of huge risks, and they paid off. I made the right choices and put my life on a far better path. Clearly, my fears of not being able to make it on my own were completely unfounded. In addition, my first foray into the law of attraction had worked, and life was fulfilling for the next number of years.

When you're on your best path in life, you tend to experience more random coincidences. Notice them. Appreciate them and keep doing what you're doing. If you've misinterpreted the guidance and taken the wrong path, don't worry: the universe will let you know by placing obstacles in your path. That's because the best paths in life are typically the paths of least resistance. If you keep experiencing multiple roadblocks on a certain path, it may be time to try other options. If you're convinced it's the right path, pause for a time and pay attention for other signs, coincidences, and synchronicity, because it may be the right path, but it's just that the timing may not have been right.

Whatever the form of guidance, we can't receive it if our connection to Home is impaired.

What Stops Us from Being Connected?

If you can't touch it, see it, or hear it, Western culture teaches us from a young age not to believe in things that we don't fully understand. This is improving over time with the help of influential people like Wayne Dyer, Deepak Chopra, Eckhart Tolle, Rhonda Byrne, and Oprah Winfrey. Many of these individuals have been able to penetrate mainstream thinking and grab the attention of those who are open to broadening their minds and belief systems.

I can also see evidence of this shift in bookstores. Twenty years ago, I'd go to the bookstore and shamefully look for reading materials in the Occult (which has very negative connotations) section. Nowadays, I proudly stroll through the Spiritual (more positive connotations) section. I'm grateful to those who have laid the path before me, because it has put more and more people in the headspace to openly receive the messages I want to convey in this book.

I expect some people may have stopped reading this book the minute they started reading my section on the trip into the blue light. That's because most of us in the Western world are taught (indirectly through conflicting messages) to shut down and ignore the channels that could keep us connected. It's a shame because, from the minute we're born, we're strongly connected to our souls. Unfortunately for most of us raised in Western culture, the connection slowly shuts down (or we start to ignore it) as we grow older and mature.

One of my earliest memories (I was three or four years old) is that of sitting alone in my grandmother's room (she lived with my family) and singing "Happy Birthday" to a picture of my late grandfather, a man I had never known, as he'd passed well before my birth. Shortly after I stopped singing, my grandmother walked in the room, and I started asking questions about the man known only to me through the picture on her dresser. She answered the questions about him, and then told me that it was his birthday.

You can imagine (even at that young of an age) how taken aback I was with the fact that I had sang to the picture only minutes earlier. I remember telling my grandmother and running to the kitchen to tell my mother. Neither one of them believed me. And so began the process of shutting down the communication channel to my soul.

You see, as infants, we're typically born with an open conduit that's tuned to the right frequency to receive guidance. Unfortunately, as we learn, grow, and become educated in Western society, the majority of us are taught that interest in things we cannot see, touch or fully understand cannot contribute to our main goals in life. We eventually learn to shut down or ignore the conduit to Home and opt for mainstream thinking. Thankfully, it's not a use-it-or-lose-it situation. Anytime we want to start paying attention, we can start putting ourselves on the path to receive messages from Home.

The primary aspects of life that cause us to ignore the connection to Home or prevent us from staying connected are the following:

1. Fear and doubt (our egos)
2. Religious beliefs
3. Emotional blockages caused by emotional trauma

Fear and Doubt

Even when the connection to Home is open and we're receiving messages loud and clear, fear and doubt prevent us from acting on the messages and making those difficult decisions to put us on our best paths in life.

When we think about the triumvirate of mind, body and soul, it's something called the *ego* that rules the mind. The mind develops and matures over time through our earthly experiences. It knows it's temporary and fleeting. I'm not an expert in psychology, but I believe Sigmund Freud first introduced the term *ego*. How I describe it in this book may not match his definition. However most of the spiritual books written today use the term *ego* to describe, on a very simple level, what governs our minds.

The ego is ever present and believes its primary purpose is to protect us. It has complete authority over our survival instincts. The ego is very aware that our existences are temporary, and since it doesn't understand the unknown, it fears death and does everything to ensure our longevity. Since a big part of survival here on earth is about food and shelter, the ego's primary goal is to focus on ensuring we have plenty to eat and roofs over our heads. It's the ego that drives us to achieve more than what we need. It's most happy when we have a steady stream of income and are protected from the elements. The ego fears any type of insecurity and instability. The ego doesn't like to take risks, particularly when it feels secure.

Our egos were designed specifically to protect us from doing something that would threaten our lives, livelihoods, and general well beings. This is beneficial when we're standing on the edge of a cliff with the wind blowing at our backs and our egos generate the fear that convinces us to step back to a safer distance. But it works against us when we've been provided with an opportunity to become self-employed and ego drives the fear that keeps us from leaving the safety of more secure employment.

Our egos have no ill intents; they don't see that they're keeping us from following our best paths in life because they truly believe they're protecting us. They're very short sighted and just want us to be safe. I'm grateful for Wayne Dyer, because pretty much every book I've read by him has a section on how to recognize and dial down the fear and doubt that's created by our egos.

With all the risks I've taken in my life, I still struggle with the fear and doubt generated by my ego, but for the most part, I've taught my ego to let go and relinquish control to the universe. I've taken enough risks and seen enough results that even my ego has learned to trust the signs, synchronicity, and guidance as I receive it. In fact, the more fear and doubt generated by my ego, the more I'm apt to push forward, explore that path a little more, and start looking for any signs of synchronicity.

> What you are afraid to do is a clear indication of the
> next thing you need to do.
> —Ralph Waldo Emerson

Religious Beliefs

Some of the concepts I present in this book conflict with the teachings of many of today's mainstream religions. Since religion is so ingrained in our culture, for many people, their religious beliefs have become part of their underlying belief (or value) system. Our value systems play very critical roles in our lives. Every day, without realizing it, whenever we make a decision or a choice, we automatically (i.e., it's an unconscious reaction) check in with our value systems to help guide our decisions and choices.

If our religious beliefs are part of our value systems that influence our life choices, then it's very easy to draw the line and understand how our religious beliefs can influence the path we take in life. It may seem counterintuitive, but holding fast to our religious beliefs can sometimes inadvertently cause us to stray from or prevent us from choosing our best path in life.

It's an unfortunate circumstance, because the act of praying to God is very similar to connecting to Home. However, when our connection to Home is shrouded in religious beliefs, we effectively reduce the capacity of the connection and the choices we can make in life. This is because we ignore the guidance we receive from Home that conflicts with our religious beliefs.

The best example I have to demonstrate this is my divorce. If I had held on to my religious beliefs, "until death do us part," I wouldn't have been on my best path in life, and I may have put my daughter's best path at risk as well. I can't say that I've completely let go of my religious beliefs, but I've certainly made adjustments to them.

I was raised in a Christian (Protestant) household. I was christened and confirmed. As a child, I attended Sunday school regularly, and in my early teens, I sang in the church choir. As I grew older, I drifted from the church in part because of time (Sundays were prime time to work when I was in university) and because my knowledge of the sciences conflicted with much of the context of the Bible. Despite that, I always envisioned returning to the church once I started a family. I had visions of reading bedtime stories about Jesus and saying bedtime prayers with my children.

After my daughter was born, I wanted to have her christened. I naively thought I could get her christened at any church. I was shocked when we were turned down by a number of churches because we weren't part of the congregation. Eventually, my aunt had to pay extra money (i.e., bribe) to have our child christened in her church. It was after that experience that I became disenchanted with Christianity and organized religion, because I could not reconcile the fact that the man who was Jesus Christ would ever have turned me or my child away.

I believe Jesus was a real person. Like Wayne Dyer or Deepak Chopra, he was a visionary and spiritual leader of his time. He was a loving and caring man who had a great positive message: "Do unto others as you would have them do unto you." He was connected to Home, and on some level, I believe he knew the principles and concepts that I've put forth in this book. However, I don't believe that he turned water into wine or parted the seas. There may have been some element of truth in these stories, but I believe they were embellished over time and that's how they were captured, when the words passed down through generations were finally written on paper.

I once read a book that caught my eye in a bookstore many years ago, called *God on a Harley*, written by Joan Brady. The premise of the book is that God comes here to earth disguised as a biker (on a Harley) and meets a woman. Over time, he gains her trust and convinces her that he never meant for religion to get out of hand like it has. He explained that humans let their egos take over religion, and as a result, humanity's belief system didn't end up the way he intended. Although that book was fiction, the overall message resonated with me.

Around the same time I read Brady's book, I also read Anthony Robbin's book *Awaken the Giant Within*, in which he helped me identify the pillars of my underlying belief system. The nuggets I took from both those books helped me uncouple many of my religious beliefs from my value system. My religious beliefs are still a big part of me, but they no longer blindly dictate my path in life. Instead of unconsciously using them to influence all my decisions, I consciously check in with them and weigh them against all other factors before I make a decision that's authentically best for me.

Although I don't subscribe to what Christianity has become, I still try to follow Jesus's do-unto-others message, and I still believe in the concept of God in that there is one source, to which we're all connected. However, I don't believe in a supreme being. Instead, I prefer to think that the universe is sentient.

Emotional Blockages

Experiencing severe emotional trauma can create emotional blockages that effectively shut down communications between here and Home. An emotional blockage is to the soul what a bacterial infection is to the body. Like most infections, an emotional blockage usually requires a professional to clear it. Emotional blockages impair our connections between here and Home. Anytime we lose the connection, we're at risk of straying off our best paths, and we also become vulnerable to the void.

For many years after the divorce, and once I became self-employed, life was rewarding and fulfilling. I was connected and living free of the void. I eventually met a wonderful man. His name was Devon, and we became lovers, confidants, and best friends. We both had children who were getting close to graduating from high school, so we decided not to blend the families and wait until the kids went to university before discussing cohabitation or any type of permanent union. For two people who didn't have good relationship track records, this decision also served as a means for us to take the relationship slowly.

Devon wasn't perfect (none of us are), but I always felt he was perfect for me. He had some mental health issues in that he struggled with anxiety and depression. When I met him, he was on medication to manage both. During the majority of our five years together, he appeared stable and happy. Even though we weren't married, he played the role of stepfather to my daughter. She adored him. Life was good for all of us. Then as the kids were making final preparations to leave home and go away to university, things quickly unravelled.

Knowing my daughter would be moving away was having a profound effect on me. I was very happy for her, but I knew I was going to miss her dearly. I didn't know what the future had in store for me. Devon's oldest son was going away to university as well. Devon, too, was struggling with letting go and moving forward. Though these struggles were having an adverse impact on our relationship, we maintained an open dialogue and were committed to working through it. We recognized we were sad about our kids leaving, but we were hopeful for our future together. For the first time in our relationship, we discussed the possibility of cohabitation and marriage.

It was also around that time that Devon decided he was unhappy with his medication because it made him drowsy during the day. To me, this wasn't an issue because he was retired, independently wealthy, and didn't have a reason to get up early. I worked full time, which meant there was little opportunity for us to spend time together during the days anyway. Besides, he was always alert in the evenings, and that's when we had our quality time together. Despite that, it made him feel like less of a person, and it bothered him enough that he decided to change his medication.

The effects of the new medication had a devastating impact on his mental health and our relationship. Within the span of three to four weeks, his personality completely changed. The man I loved became someone else. He broke up with me about six days after the kids left for university. This was incomprehensible to me. At the time, I thought he was having a midlife crisis. I've since learned that the change in medication triggered a manic episode.

Not recognizing the full gravity of the situation and the depth of his mental health issues, my mind wasn't equipped to fully process such a sudden breakup. I shut down emotionally. Outwardly at the time, it appeared to my friends that I had little or no reaction to the event. Inwardly, I buried all the feelings (anger, crushing heartbreak, betrayal) and pushed forward with life. In the back of my mind, I hoped he would work through (what I thought was) his midlife crisis and we'd eventually get back together.

There is a saying: when one door closes, another one opens. In between those six days, after the kids left for university and when Devon broke up with me, I received a phone call from a former client asking if I wanted to take a contract with him in Minneapolis. If I didn't have such strong spiritual beliefs, I'd have ignored the opportunity in Minneapolis and stayed in Nova Scotia and monitored Devon's situation. However, the fact that those two events happened so close together was a sign for me. I interpreted it as a strong form of guidance and synchronicity, and I graciously walked through that open door, accepted the contract, and (for the time being) let the door on my life with Devon close behind me.

Looking back now, and hearing about Devon's out-of-character actions during the time I was in Minnesota, staying in eastern Canada would have been very difficult for me. Instead, I felt as if the universe gently picked me up, insulated me, and put me in a safe place so I wouldn't be affected by his activities during that time.

I loved living in Minnesota. It always felt magical to me, but when my daughter was coming home from university the following summer, I wanted to be with her. I returned home eight months after Devon broke up with me. After I was settled back in eastern Canada, I began to consider if I should reach out to him. I'd heard through mutual friends he wasn't doing well. But I never got the opportunity. Shortly thereafter, Devon took his own life.

Because there had been an eight-month gap from the time we'd broken up until Devon passed away, I didn't feel I had the right to grieve him. Once again, I buried my emotions and pushed forward with life. I've since learned that you don't get to choose who or how you grieve someone, and there's a very big price to pay for suppressing (not expressing) emotions. Eighteen months after his death, my emotional state had degraded to the point where my normal coping skills were no longer effective.

Since I hadn't properly processed the emotional fallout from the breakup, or his death, I had created an emotional blockage. I was no longer able to connect to Home, and for the second time in my life, I was stuck, frozen, and paralyzed. I was feeling the void again. Through discussions with my doctor and counselor, I decided to take some time off work. I knew my soul was sick again, but this time, I knew how to heal it.

I took five months off work to focus on my soul's health. I traveled to visit friends and family in western Canada and the United States. It was during that time that I went on another retreat in Sedona. Once again, I worked with an amazing group of practitioners to help me connect with and heal my soul. They cleared the emotional blockages. It was during this retreat that I had my second experience with Home, and was offered a glimpse of what my soul really looks like. It was also there that I made a commitment to leverage the law of attraction again, and I set new intentions for my life. I wanted to become an author and write a book.

After I left Sedona, I felt lighter, recharged, and grounded, and I started pondering about writing a book. It's always been something I've felt compelled to do, but I had no clue how or where to start.

Then about a week after my trip to Sedona, I woke up one morning at five thirty, and I had an idea for my book. I immediately picked up my journal and started writing. I continued to write for the next ninety minutes. The ideas just kept coming. A lot of what I was writing didn't make sense to me at the time, but I dismissed the urge to start questioning what I was doing and I just kept writing. I suspected I was being guided, as I felt this continual flow of energy coming through me.

At one point, I even remember thinking, *This is really good stuff. I'm going to have to do some research.* Then I got a clear and distinct message that said, *No research is required. You are the expert.* Since that isn't something I'd say to myself, it was complete confirmation that this was guidance. I shut down my ego, brushed aside any doubt, tuned into the stream of consciousness, and kept writing. Furiously.

> My brain is only a receiver, in the universe there is a
> core from which we obtain knowledge, strength and
> inspiration. I have not penetrated into the secrets of
> this core, but I know that it exists.
>
> —Nikola Tesla

I'm not sure how I was able to maintain the connection for so long. Perhaps it was because I had been meditating at least ten minutes a day for the prior three months. Or perhaps that early in the morning, when the energy generated by people commuting to work is absent, there is less interference, and it's much easier to tune in. There is a quote by Rumi: "The breeze at dawn has secrets to tell you. Don't go back to sleep." I'm so grateful I reached for my journal that morning.

Clearly, my second retreat in Sedona was successful, and my emotional blockages had been cleared. The content generated from the stream of consciousness that morning became the foundation for this book. I finally had a place to start.

Conclusion

Our souls are our true selves, and the energy of the universe that surrounds all living things provides us with opportunities to communicate with our souls while we're here on earth. We can leverage that communication to improve our lives by understanding the following:

1. Each of us has a unique journey on this earth, a well-planned path laid out before us.
2. We have free will and the ability to make our own choices, which can keep us on our best paths in life or cause us to stray from them.
3. The closer we are to our best path, the more fulfilling and rewarding life is.
4. Our souls understand our best paths and can help us navigate there.
5. Fear, doubt, religion, and emotional blockages are some of the main barriers that prevent us from connecting with our souls and cause us to ignore guidance from them.

6. Straying from the path can lead to feelings of unfulfillment, depression, and eventually even suicidal thoughts.
7. As a result of emotional trauma, our souls can become ill, which can hinder our abilities to receive guidance.
8. Similar to our minds and bodies, we must also care for and heal our souls, as they're crucial to our emotional, mental, and physical well beings.

Not only do we receive guidance to place us on our best paths, but also some of us are being guided to communicate about how we can connect with our souls, through many different mediums including books, podcasts, and movies. Certainly, the idea that one energy field surrounds and supports us all is very similar to the concept of the Force in George Lucas's epic Star Wars saga.

The concepts described in this book are not new and have been around for centuries. It's my hope that all sources (fiction and non-fiction), will eventually create a shift in the minds of (wo)men and reach a tipping point where these ideas and concepts will become mainstream.

Section 2

Staying Connected by Taking Care of Your Soul

Staying connected to Home sets us up to receive the guidance that can keep us on our best paths and lead us to more fulfilling lives. In order to receive clear communication from Home, not only do we need to stay connected, but also the energy from Home must be able to flow freely around and through us. If the energy around us is not flowing freely, our souls can lose their connection to Home. The intent of this section is to help you understand how to promote the free flow of energy around you by nurturing, feeding, and caring for your soul.

Everything Is Energy—Part 2

Just like everything else in the universe, humans are surrounded by an energy field. Sometimes called an *aura* or an *energetic body*, it's part of the system our souls use to connect with Home. In fact, our souls and energy fields are so tightly integrated, that when we care for our souls, we're also caring for our energy fields and vice versa.

The inherent problem with staying connected is that the energy from Home vibrates at a much higher frequency than the energy levels here on earth. The energy levels here on earth are thick and slow, and vibrate at a very low level. While energy levels at Home vibrate at very high levels and are light and airy. The lower the vibration in our energy fields, the more out of sync we are with the energy from Home and the less likely we are to be able to connect and stay connected.

Unfortunately, from the minute we're born (when our connection to Home is the strongest), we become surrounded by circumstances and environmental conditions that can lower the vibrations in our energy fields or create "interference." Similar to the static we experience when we're not quite tuned in to a radio station, interference in our energy fields can garble the messages and make it difficult to receive the guidance from Home.

Understanding how to manage and counteract the effects of interference and lower vibrations is critical to staying connected to Home. There are many things that can create interference, lower our vibration and inhibit the free flow of energy around us. In fact, some of the worst offenders are our own thoughts and emotions. This is because, thoughts and emotions, are just another form of energy.

> "If you want to find the secrets of the universe, think
> in terms of energy, frequency and vibration."
> —Nikola Tesla

The Power of Thought

Thoughts are one of the most powerful sources of energy in the universe. Whenever a thought pops into our heads, it naturally integrates with the energy that flows through and around us.

When it comes to thoughts, there are two absolute truths:

- Positive thoughts raise your vibration and promote a healthy flow of energy around you.
- Negative thoughts lower your vibration and cause interference that can hinder the free flow of energy around you.

When the connection to Home is clearer and more free flowing, positive thoughts are not just able to enter your energy field, but they're also more likely to intermingle with the energy of the collective conscience. This is how the magic of coincidences and synchronicity can happen. Thinking of someone and having them call you shortly thereafter is a good indicator your energy is free flowing and you have a good connection to Home.

A positive and healthy energy field isn't only the foundation for establishing a clear conduit with Home; it's also a key element in the law of attraction. The simplest definition of the law of attraction is that you attract what you are. If your energy field is positive, you'll attract positivity into your life. If your energy field is negative, you'll attract negativity into your life. Left unchecked, negative thoughts can also lead to feeling the void.

Wayne Dyer wrote a book called *Change Your Thoughts—Change Your Life*. From that book I learned that in the split second before we hold a thought, we have the opportunity to choose it. This gives us the power to select a positive thought over a negative one. When I read that book many years ago, it resonated with me, and I made it my mission to slowly and methodically change the way I think about everything.

With my less-than-ideal upbringing, through adolescence and into early adulthood, my thought patterns were rooted in negativity. When my mother wasn't physically abusing me, she was berating me and my character (even as a small toddler). This created a near constant stream of negative thoughts in my head. My one saving grace was that I always did well in school. I chose to let that define me, and I did my best to focus on that aspect of my character and tune out the negative influence of my mother.

As I became a young adult, I knew I didn't want to be like my mother, but I didn't know or understand the alternatives. Thankfully, after I earned my degree and entered the workforce, I met many strong female role models. It was refreshing, eye opening, and life changing for me, as I started modeling their positive behaviors and eliminating my negative ones.

I can't pinpoint the exact time my energy field changed from positive to negative. For me, changing the nature of my thought patterns was a journey, and my success has been a result of receiving good counseling, reading many self-help books, and adapting my behaviors to match those of positive role models. Although I can still get dragged into the negative headspace that my mother created for me, for the most part, it's natural for me to choose positive thoughts.

> I am not what happened to me. I am what I choose
> to become.
>
> —C. G. Jung

One of the many benefits of turning my thought patterns from negative to positive is that I can now see the silver lining in just about any situation. Although the abuse I suffered as a child was difficult to endure, the silver lining is that it has made me resilient and determined as an adult. This resiliency has helped me cope (in particular) with the emotional pain I suffered after my divorce and in coming to terms with Devon's death.

There is no doubt that thoughts have the power to change your life, and there are some forms of thought that are more powerful than others.

Powerful Forms of Thought

Intentions—Put simply, intentions are thoughts with purposes. Formed and delivered correctly, your intentions can permeate your energy field, the collective conscience, and actually direct the universe how to support you in life. Setting intentions is also a foundational aspect of the law of attraction.

Affirmations—Affirmations are like intentions, but they're not quite as personalized. They're positive thoughts that can organize the energy of the universe around you. Saying affirmations is a good way to start your day and to get you thinking positively from the outset.

Prayer—Most of us equate prayer with religion because that's where we learned how to pray. Prayer is organized thought that can have positive affects on your energy field. As long as the content of a prayer is positive toward you, other people, or the universe, it'll promote and foster the healthy flow of energy around you and the object of your prayers.

Although I haven't practiced traditional religion in a long time, I still pray, but I no longer recite traditional prayers I learned in church.

Instead, I close my eyes, hold feelings of love and gratitude, and pray for the healing of unhealthy situations in my life, the earth, and other people.

By praying for another person, not only will you raise your vibration, but also you'll stand a good chance of raising the vibration of the person you're praying for. This can be more effective if the person's thought patterns aren't rooted in negativity. If the person's energy field is negative, slow, and thick, your prayers may do little to impact them. However, I never take that into consideration when I pray for someone else. If I feel someone needs support from the universe, I'll pray for them and hope that others are praying for them too. This is where the power of prayer has its highest potential, as many people praying for one person can raise the vibration of the person in need.

One of the reasons thoughts are so powerful is that they can produce strong emotions.

The Power of Emotion

Emotions are powerful for two very simple reasons:

- Negative thoughts tend to produce and amplify negative emotions that lower your vibration and create interference.
- Positive thoughts tend to produce and amplify positive emotions that raise your vibration and reduce or eliminate interference.

Sometimes emotions can be temporary, while other times emotions can consume us and even define who we are. The same negative emotion experienced over a long period of time can go from just causing interference (i.e., make it difficult to connect to Home) to an emotional blockage (i.e., make it almost impossible to connect to Home).

Similar to thoughts, emotions also have the power to change our lives. And some emotions are more powerful than others.

Powerful Emotions

The list of powerful emotions is endless. I list the following because they're the emotions that I've struggled with the most in life.

Love—Love is the purest of all emotions and is the essence of the energy that flows around, through us, and between here and Home. When we're born, we're pure little beings of love, having full potential to love and to be loved. Holding and expressing feelings of love toward others will help raise your vibration and the vibration of the individual(s) who is (or are) receiving your affection.

Self-Love—Self-love is the platform/foundation on which positive thoughts and emotions can grow. It's like fertilizer for positive thoughts/emotions. Where there's no self-love, feelings of self-loathing can amplify other negative thoughts and emotions, which will lower your vibration and create interference. It can become a vicious cycle.

I spent much of my life feeling no self-love. I don't remember the day I woke up and decided I liked the person looking back at me in the mirror. It just seemed to happen naturally as I eliminated negative thought patterns, cleared emotional blockages, and received good therapy. My path to self-discovery and self-acceptance was a long journey. I love who I am today, and the sense of pride I feel about myself makes me grateful for all the experiences (good and bad) in my life.

Gratitude—Holding feelings of gratitude is like planting little magnets in your field of energy. It tells the universe what you want to attract into your life. Holding feelings of gratitude is also very important to the law of attraction. Once you set your intentions, gratitude is the best way to reinforce them and remind the universe about the things you want more of. Whenever I'm experiencing a pleasant situation (i.e., something I want more of), I pause, savor the moment, and feel very grateful.

Worrying—Similar to gratitude, the act of worrying also plants little magnets in your field of energy, except instead of attracting more of what we want, worrying attracts more of what we don't want. Worrying is a powerful negative emotion that serves no useful purpose in our lives. It's a habit that can be broken with focused effort and attention. I say this because at one time I was a chronic worrier.

Shame—Shame is an emotion that is put upon us by others. As children, we learned to survive by adapting and following the family unit values system (which likely included religious beliefs and cultural and social norms). If guidance from our souls, is not aligned with our family values, then we can feel like who we are, is wrong or bad. One of the reasons I wrote this book was because I've witnessed my friends struggle with their shame and their soul's desire to choose a better path forward. This constant conflict between who we really are, and who others say we should be, can lower our vibration and make us vulnerable to feeling the void.

Being able to move forward peacefully on our best path, may mean eliminating and/or reducing the sources of shame in our lives. This can be difficult (but not impossible), if it's someone we love. Making the decision to be authentically true to ourselves, is a good place to start.

Guilt—Guilt is another wasted emotion that creates interference in our energy field and lowers our vibration. Whereas shame is put upon us by others, we invite guilt into our lives and energy fields, when we do something that goes against our underlying value systems. Understanding the makeup of our own value system and identifying and letting go of the constructs (e.g., religious beliefs, unrealistic family expectations, outdated social norms) that are not aligned with our soul, can go a long way in removing the sources of guilt in our lives.

Grief—When I studied introductory psychology in university 35 years ago, I learned that we experience grief in five stages: denial, anger, bargaining, depression and acceptance. This suggests that processing grief is a linear experience. However, while coming to terms with Devon's death, I discovered that grief is actually a cyclical experience. In fact, more recent research indicates that after we lose a loved one, even though initially we may experience the five stages, as time passes, we may also suffer setbacks that will cause us to revert back through one or more of the stages. My setbacks (during which I can go through all the stages in one day), typically occur on special occasions and anniversaries that I shared with Devon. How we experience grief is a personal experience and differs for everyone.

In addition, it is important to note that grief it is not just associated with the death of a loved one. Greif can be experienced any time we suffer a major loss in our lives. This can include the loss of a relationship (i.e., divorce), a job, a way of life or even the loss of a body part (through accident or life saving surgery). Regardless of the root cause, unprocessed grief causes interference and creates emotional blockages in our energy fields. For me, becoming aware of the cyclical nature of grief, and making the choice to be with my emotions instead of suppressing them, finally helped me move forward in peace.

Stress and Anxiety—There's a long list of powerful negative emotions that can hinder the flows of energy, lower our vibrations, and even cause emotional blockages. In addition, when negative thoughts and emotions get overwhelming, they have the power to amplify feelings of stress and anxiety, which not only affects your ability to connect with Home, but also can adversely impact your mental and physical health.

Negative thoughts and negative emotions are not the only things that can lower your vibration. There are certain behaviors and activities that will lower your vibration and cause interference. I've listed some of the more common ones below.

Behaviors/Activities That Lower Your Vibration

Most people who engage in behaviors that lower vibration do so because they're either trying to fill the void or mask negative emotions or their energy fields are vibrating at such a low level (likely caused by past trauma) that they continue low-level behaviors because that's what they're comfortable with. It becomes a vicious cycle that can be difficult to escape.

Substance Abuse—Prolonged abuse of alcohol, illegal or prescription drugs and/or food (i.e., emotional eating) will lower vibration and inhibit the free flow of energy around you. This isn't because drugs/food contain negative energy, but it's typically because over time these activities tend to produce feelings of regret, guilt, shame, remorse, and self-loathing, which amplify and lead to more negative thoughts and emotions.

Abusing Others—Any act of physical or emotional abuse (including controlling, manipulating, and bullying) against another person has an adverse effect on both individuals. As negative emotions and thoughts from the abuser permeate the field of the person being abused, they essentially lower the vibration of each person and create ongoing interference for both individuals.

Violent Criminal Behavior—The act(s) of an intentional violent crime has detrimental effects on both the perpetrators and the victims. Assuming the victim survives, it's more than likely they may have been traumatized by the violent act(s). This of course will create emotional blockages that can greatly impair their connection to Home. However, the effects on the perpetrator are more detrimental because the strength of the emotions that led to the crime(s) could be so strong that the perpetrator's vibration may be lowered to a point where they may shut down their connections to Home.

Toxic People—Spending time (or even just communicating) with people who are rooted in negativity will lower your vibration and create interference in your energy field. If you have toxic people in your life, keep your interactions (this includes phone, email, text) to a minimum to avoid the adverse impact they can have on your energy field and (ultimately) the quality of your life.

If you're engaging in any of these behaviors and can't eliminate them on your own, it's important to seek professional help (preferably from practitioners who understand both the mind and the soul) and receive treatment/rehabilitation. Otherwise, you may find yourself spiraling downward, feeling the void and unable to connect with Home.

Fortunately, there are many ways to raise your vibration and clear interference in your energy field. Practicing and making self-care a priority in your life is one of the most effective ways to manage interference and promote a healthy flow of energy. The next section describes some of the more common methods that I use to take care of myself. Establishing a regular self-care regimen is an individual pursuit, and most people need to spend time discovering (i.e., research methods not in this book) and experimenting with what makes their souls happy.

Managing Interference and Raising Your Vibration through Self-Care

Self-care aimed at feeding and nourishing your soul on a daily basis will foster positive thoughts and emotions, raise your vibration, detoxify your energy field, and keep your connection to Home clear of static. In developing your own self-care regime, I recommend (if you haven't already) trying some of the activities listed below or perhaps try them again with a new perspective. In developing your own self-care regimen, be bold and adventurous.

Meditation—For a long time my perception of meditating was a group of monks, sitting in stillness and trying to empty their minds of all thought. Over time however, I've broadened my definition, and

I now realize that meditation is just as much about being mindful (or mindfulness) as it is about emptying the mind.

For me, the practice of meditating on a regular basis is trying to focus on one thing (usually the breath). And the objective of meditating, it isn't to empty the mind of all thought, but to train the mind to catch itself when it decides to wander. Along with quieting your mind, this has the added benefit of increasing your awareness of your thought patterns, such that in daily life, you can be more aware of that split second when you decide to choose a positive thought, instead of a negative one.

The other key to a good meditation practice, isn't to judge or berate yourself when your mind wanders. This will defeat the purpose of meditating, as it generates negative thought. Be grateful for that moment when you catch your mind wandering, it means you just did one more repetition to exercise that part of your brain, that will help you choose and maintain positive thought patterns.

Another benefit of meditation is that your mind is a little less busy after you finish a session, which makes it one of the best times to pose specific questions to the universe and listen for any guidance/ messages from Home.

Establishing a meditation practice is an important part of maintaining a healthy soul and energy field. Whether you choose guided, unguided, or both forms of meditations, it doesn't matter. The key is to dedicate whatever time you can spare (even if it's only ten minutes a day) on a regular basis.

Yoga—Yoga isn't only good for the soul; it also benefits the mind and the body. In fact, the objective of most yoga practices is to align your mind, body and soul.

I personally struggled with my yoga practice for many years. I could see my friends and family enjoying it, but every time I attended a class, I walked away feeling worse than I went in. Recently, I read a book called *The Empath's Survival Guide*, written by Dr. Judith Orloff, that explained why I was feeling that way. I discovered I'm an "empath" (a person who's capable of feeling and absorbing other people's energy). Since one of the objectives of yoga is releasing toxic negative energy, instead of releasing my negative energy in large classes, I was absorbing everyone else's. I've since been able to establish my own yoga practice at home, and on occasion, I will join a small class with others when I want to improve my technique.

There are many other forms of exercise (e.g., tai chi, qigong) that promote a healthy flow of energy. I encourage you to experiment with them all and adopt a practice that works best for you.

Time in Nature—Trees, flowers, plants, birds, and even insects exude positive energy. Spending time in nature, skiing, snowboarding, snowshoeing, walking, jogging, hiking, biking, kayaking or any other activity you enjoy outside, will allow positive energy from the natural elements to permeate and raise the vibration of your energy field.

Putting your hands in soil (gardening) or walking on grass/sand in your bare feet is a great way to rid your body of negative energy, absorb positive energy from the earth and raise your vibration.

Bathing—Bathing in water is a natural detoxifier, and bathing in water that has been infused with Epsom salts (or even better, the ocean) can help raise your vibration and reduce interference.

Essential Oils—Essential oils carry their own vibrations, and using them for their intended purposes can alter moods/emotions and raise your vibration.

Music—There is music, and then there is the kind of music that touches and resonates with your soul. I have very eclectic taste in music. I don't listen to any particular genre. But there are certain songs that just tickle my insides. If listening to certain music does that for you too, then do your best to keep that music as a background in your daily life to help promote a healthy flow of energy around you.

If you're someone who plays an instrument or sings (especially if the music is coming from your soul), the effects of creating music can be more powerful than just listening to it. Playing music or singing on your own, or with a group of like-minded souls, is a very effective means to reduce interference, raise your vibration, and keep your energy free flowing.

Hobbies—Any type of hobby or activity that stimulates the creative centers in your brain will help connect you with the energy of Home, raise your vibration, and reduce interference.

Time with Soul Mates—Most people's perspective on the term *soul mate* is that it's an intimate partner and that we're limited to only one in our lifetime. That's not the case, as we can have any number of friends (and even family members) who can be considered soul mates. A soul mate is just someone with whom you feel a very special connection (i.e., your energy fields are compatible) and who just generally makes you feel better when you're in their presence. Time spent with a soul mate will reduce interference and help raise the vibration of both individuals.

Orgasm—Orgasm is one of the most enjoyable ways to raise your vibration and reduce interference. However, the benefits from having an orgasm can be greatly reduced depending on the relationship you have with your sexual partner. This is because when you have sex with someone, your energy fields intermingle. If you're having sex with a loving partner, then the energy exchange between you will most likely be healthy and will benefit the both of you. If you're having sex in the absence of love, you're putting yourself at risk of possibly absorbing your partner's negative energy (similar to a sexually transmitted disease for the body), which can reduce any benefits you may gain from an orgasm.

The effects of orgasm through masturbation can have the same positive effects as with a partner, unless you feel guilt or shame afterward, at which point, you would likely counteract any benefit from the self-achieved orgasm.

Healing the Earth—Other than places like Sedona, the energy flows around the earth can become cluttered with interference created by all the discourse (e.g., wars, terrorism) in today's society. This inadvertently impacts our energy fields as well. So it's just as important to take steps to heal our planet in addition to ourselves. Through meditation you can spend a little time each day, helping to raise the vibration of the energy of the earth. This will raise your vibration and reduce interference in your field as well.

My daily self-care regimen consists of the following:

Morning

- five-minute meditation for healing the earth
- recite daily affirmations
- fifteen minutes of yoga
- guided (I use an app on my phone) meditation (ten minutes)

Throughout the Day

- pause and hold feelings of gratitude for any situation/ experience I'd like to repeat/attract into my life
- diffuse essential oils
- listen to music that feeds my soul

Evenings

- journal my thoughts on the day and any coincidences that happened during the day
- fifteen minutes of yoga (relaxation focused)
- pray (I usually hold a feeling of love and gratitude, and I pray for people and unhealthy situations in my life to be healed. I also pray for anyone who I feel needs support from Home.)

Some people think (as I once did) that taking time for yourself is selfish. I've since learned that the exact opposite it true. In moderation, practicing self-care is very similar to the messaging we receive when we're on an airplane and the flight attendant tells us to place our own oxygen mask on first, before we assist others. Self-care ensures we're healthy and can infuse positive energy toward the people who depend on us most.

Maximizing Opportunities to Connect to Home

The more we're connected to Home, the more likely we are to receive the guidance that will put us on our best path and help us lead more fulfilling lives. It makes sense then that one of our goals in life should be to create as many opportunities to connect to Home as possible.

We all come here with at least one (some are blessed with many) special skill/talent that connects us to Home and our soul. Whenever we use our special skills, we inherently raise our vibrations and connect with Home. If the path to fulfillment is finding as many opportunities to connect as possible, then the more we use our special talents, the more we're connecting to Home. Although it's not always possible and practical, the ideal situation would be to use your special talents regularly during the execution of your job/vocation, as this situation typically sets you up with the most opportunities to connect.

Some find it easier to discover their special talent than others. What I've observed through personal experience and watching others is that when people are using their special talent, they're either creating something or helping others or both.

I've spent thirty-two years as an IT professional and started out my career as a computer programmer. On the surface, it wouldn't appear that working with computers would connect me with my soul. However, when I was developing code early in my career, I'd get lost and completely lose track of time (a sure sign you're connected to Home). That's because, I've since realized, I *was* creating! I wasn't creating something beautiful like a painting or music. I was creating and designing business applications. Not only that, but also I was helping others, and I derived great satisfaction from developing applications that made other people's work lives easier.

As I progressed through my career, I eventually moved away from programming and into middle management. Looking back, that's also when I started losing job satisfaction and no longer enjoyed my work. Management is about motivating and understanding what makes people tick. It's about creating a positive environment for people to thrive. That's not to say that being a manager isn't someone else's special talent. It just wasn't mine. I quickly left management to become a consultant.

As a consultant, I found great pleasure and fulfillment in helping my clients be successful. But when I really felt the free flow of energy, when I'd get lost in the moment, was when I was writing. Having a concept come together in my mind and finding the right words/images to build the sentences and the diagrams to convey the message fed my soul.

Throughout my professional life while I was writing computer code to develop a business application or writing business documents to capture and convey a corporate message or strategy, I was unknowingly honing my special skill as a writer. Through those efforts, I learned how to absorb information from many different sources and synthesize it all to create a message and clearly communicate it to an intended audience.

I've only recently realized (as I write this book) that I applied those same skills over several years to synthesize information I gleaned from books, counselors, practitioners, and my spiritual experiences to develop the concepts I'm writing about in this book.

If you haven't identified your special talent yet, I suggest you start by trying to identify the moments in your life when you completely lost track of time and couldn't possibly think of doing anything else. If you're able to pinpoint those moments, think about the skill (not the job title or what you were producing) you were using at that time.

It's important to think at the skill level because some skills can be used across many different jobs. If you're not finding enough opportunities to use your special skill in your current job, then perhaps finding another job can produce other ways to utilize your talents and will provide you with more opportunities to connect and find fulfilment.

If it's a very specialized skill, and changing jobs isn't an option, then perhaps you can make a conscious effort to place more priority on using your special talent more often throughout your day. If you're not able to use your special talent during the execution of your job, then the next best strategy is to use it as much as possible in your spare time.

Using your skills and talents not only helps you stay connected but also feeds your soul and combats interference. When interference created by the daily stresses of life or emotional blockages from past trauma can't be managed through a self-care regimen, or you don't have time in your busy life to maintain your energy field, there are additional methods and trained practitioners who can help you.

Using Professionals/Practitioners to Help Connect You with Home

Listed below are some of the many types of practitioners and methods I've leveraged to clear interference, reduce the effects of emotional blockages and boost my connection to Home.

Reiki—Reiki is to the soul what massage therapy is to the body. Similar to a massage therapist, a certified Reiki practitioner can work with your energy field to help reduce blockages, clear interference, or just perform a tune up to promote a healthy flow in your energy field.

Although, I obtained my Reiki certification many years ago, I've never developed a Reiki practice. During my training, I was amazed how I could actually feel a person's energy field and sense how negative energy felt heavy, while positive energy felt very light.

Chakra Clearing—As humans we have seven chakras attached to our energy fields. The chakras are the main entry/exit points as energy flows in and around our bodies. Since emotional blockages can occur at the chakra openings, keeping our chakras clear (something we can either do by ourselves or through a practitioner) can promote a healthier flow of energy in your field.

Counseling/Therapy—I wouldn't be the person I am today without the help of my counselor. When thinking of the mind, body and soul, counseling is something that's typically associated with the mind. However, recognizing the strong link between thoughts and emotions and their potential to impact our connection to Home, it becomes just as necessary to treat the mind, because it can reduce interference that stems from negative thought patterns and our own mental health issues.

I was very fortunate because my counselor's belief system is similar to mine. He treats not just the mind, but the soul as well. Finding the right therapist can be difficult. Most people will ask for a recommendation from their family doctor. I found my therapist through a recommendation from a friend. If someone you like and respect, is having success with a particular therapist, chances are, you may have success with that therapist too.

Angel Therapy Practitioners—If you're struggling to connect with Home, there are individuals whose special skill is tuning into the energy of the universe and filtering out the chaos. These talented people are called Angel Therapy Practitioners (ATPs). They have the ability to see beyond our emotional blockages and interference and can receive guidance from Home on our behalf. In a sense, they boost the signal for us. ATPs can help guide us onto our best life paths, clear our energy fields and pinpoint the parts of our lives that may be causing interference or blockages.

At one point in history, these people may have been referred to as psychics, a word that typically holds negative connotations in mainstream thinking. However, angel therapy is becoming a well-recognized field. I've had sessions with both psychics and ATPs. The biggest difference I can see between them comes down to their interpretation of the messages they receive on your behalf. I've found that psychics tend to interpret the messages before they pass it on to you, whereas an ATP is trained not to judge or interpret the messages. A good ATP will tell you exactly what they're seeing or hearing, and then they'll work with you to help you decipher and interpret the message(s).

I was introduced to an ATP about fifteen years ago. Being someone whose energy field was clogged and cluttered most of my life, she was instrumental in helping me connect with Home and guiding me onto my best path several times. Through her, I also gained confidence and learned to trust my own ability to receive and interpret guidance from Home.

It's important to know that you and your ATP don't need to be in the same physical location. I usually connect with my ATP over the phone. Since we're all connected to Home, we're all essentially connected to one another. This allows ATPs to tune in to our energies and be effective, wherever they are.

Before I make a major decision in my life, I always check in with her. However, just like any other professionals, ATPs have good days and bad days, which is why I don't blindly follow all the advice I receive. I always use common sense before I make a choice and move forward on my path.

For many years I felt compelled to write a book and discussed it with my ATP on several occasions. She always indicated that it wasn't the right time. My desire to write was so strong that on a few occasions, I started writing books anyway. Unfortunately, I could never finish them, as I could never quite decide the book's purpose or the messages I wanted to convey.

After I started writing this book, I checked in with my ATP again. The first thing she said in the session (before I even asked about writing a book) was "I understand you've started a new project. It's very important, and you have to finish it." Looking back at my unfinished manuscripts, I realize now that I didn't have all the information I needed to write a comprehensive book until the stream of consciousness happened shortly after my last trip to Sedona.

Through my ATP, I also learned the value of using Oracle cards and angel numbers as other sources to help validate and interpret guidance from Home on those days when my head is filled with earthly thoughts and worries (i.e., interference).

Oracle Cards—You can purchase these cards from any reputable bookstore. If you don't have access to a bookstore, they can be purchased online. However, I find picking the right deck of cards (there are several different types) is a personal choice and best accomplished by physically looking at and touching the boxes to find a set that speaks to you.

Oracle cards are specifically designed to facilitate and interpret guidance and advice from Home. As part of my nightly routine, I draw a card and then journal my interpretation. I took a course from my ATP and learned how to work with the cards, but most decks come with an instruction booklet, so you can learn how to use and interpret them yourself.

Angel Numbers—I have a book of angel numbers that I reference on a regular basis. Before I consult the book, I clear my mind and let a number pop in. When I hear the number, I refer to the book and read the guidance associated with that number.

If you've tried some/all of these methods and are still not able to connect to Home by yourself, you may have an emotional blockage that regular maintenance activities cannot clear. In these instances, your soul may be sick, and you may require a trained practitioner to heal it and your connection to Home.

> Sleep doesn't help if it's your soul that's tired.
>
> —Unknown

Powerful Healing Treatments for the Soul

The following are some of the ways I've worked with trained practitioners to heal my soul.

Personalized Spiritual Retreats

This section is one of the main reasons I felt compelled to write this book. If your soul has been traumatized, if you've tried everything listed above, and are still feeling the void, depressed, and despairing, you'll likely need assistance from an experienced practitioner and a concentrated dose of energy from Home to help heal your soul. A spiritual retreat can do that for you.

Sedona isn't the only place you can go on a spiritual retreat, but it's the only place I've ever needed to go. Any work performed by a practitioner (located in Sedona) will be amplified and supported by the energy there.

Healing the soul can only be performed by an experienced practitioner. I've used the word *practitioner* because (although there is movement in this direction) there doesn't seem to be a well-recognized designation for those gifted people who heal the soul. I've had the honor and pleasure of meeting several of these people, and the one thing they have in common is that they all started out life in the mainstream but eventually felt a calling to use their special skill(s) to heal the soul.

I believe the reason there is no professional designation for these people is because there are so many different methods, means and modalities to heal our souls. Some practitioners use sound (e.g., musical instruments and chanting), others use discussion methods (similar to counselors), while still others use guided meditation. Regardless of their skills and methods, they can be very effective in healing the parts of our souls that prevent us from connecting to Home.

Spiritual retreats can be expensive to attend individually. Group retreats are less expensive, but they're not tailored to you. If you feel you need a personalized experience and can't afford it, plant an intention and let the universe find a way to take you there.

Just like any profession, some practitioners (who heal the soul) are better than others. It may take some time to find one that's right for you. If you set the right intention and work in tandem with the universe, you'll be guided to the individual(s) who can help you because, not surprisingly, there are people whose special skill is to match you up with the right practitioner.

Soul Retrieval

Throughout this book I have made reference to the fact that the soul can become ill or sick. That's not technically accurate, but it's a good analogy and is an easy way to describe what can happen to our souls after we experience a traumatizing event. Instead of using the terms sick or ill, it's more accurate to say that trauma can affect us either by creating emotional blockages in our energy fields or by causing pieces (or all) of our souls to separate (or fragment) from our bodies. In fact, when a person uses the term "out of body experience" to describe an event in their life, they quite likely are referring to a time when they felt their soul leave their body. A fragmented soul has gaps that inhibit the free flow of energy around the body. These gaps can only be repaired by an experienced practitioner.

I've experienced a couple of sessions during which a practitioner pulled back the orphaned pieces of my soul. These sessions, referred to as *soul retrieval*, can be quite powerful. During my last trip to Sedona, a practitioner brought me out on the famous red rocks, where I lay on the ground with the energy from Home flowing all around me. He then used many techniques and implements, including drumming, chimes, chanting, affirmations and a didgeridoo, to interact with the energy in my field and call the orphaned pieces of my soul back to me.

Even though my eyes were closed, I could see the red rocks of Sedona in my mind, just as if I were a bird in flight. Then I started to recognize the bits of my soul as they returned. Prior to the session, I'd thought the holes in my soul were only caused by Devon's death, but I was amazed at how many other of my past experiences had caused my soul to separate.

After the lost pieces of my soul returned, I felt my soul celebrating the reunion. It was at that time I had my second experience (as I recounted in Section 1) with Home and saw my soul (that beautiful glowing crystal of light and energy).

My soul-retrieval sessions have taught me that most of us may not be aware of all the experiences that have caused us emotional trauma. Sometimes trauma is obvious, such as when someone is a victim of violent crime. While other times, as in my situation, it may be masked. I spent the first thirty-five years of my life not recognizing that my abusive upbringing traumatized me. We need to keep an open mind when we look back through our pasts and try to identify what is causing our emotional pain in the present.

It's crucial to note that we're all individuals, and we all react to situations and circumstances differently. What may cause emotional trauma in one person, may not affect another as deeply. How we handle emotional trauma is unique to each of us, so it's important not to compare or judge ourselves for the way we've been affected by trauma. In addition, past trauma tends to weaken an individual's energy field, making those who've been traumatized early in life more susceptible to being affected when they experience potentially traumatizing events as adults.

Forgiveness

Forgiving someone is one of the hardest things to do, but it's one of the most freeing and powerful things you can do *for yourself.* Grudges and feelings of anger and resentment toward others are negative emotions that permeate and inhibit the flow of *your energy.* They have *no impact* on the energy field of the other person. Prolonged feelings of anger and resentment can even create emotional blockages. That's why it's best to do whatever you can to forgive those who have wronged you.

Forgiveness can be most powerful when we tell the individual(s) in person that we forgive them, but it's not necessary. This is because forgiveness is really about finding a way to let go of the negative emotions we feel toward the individual(s), and we don't need to interact with the person(s) in order to accomplish that.

Sometimes we find it difficult to forgive someone (especially if they haven't apologized to us) because it feels as though they're getting away with something. We may perceive them as never being "punished" for their actions. However, it's important to take a step back and look at the situation from a broader perspective. When someone truly harms (emotionally or physically) another person, the effect of those actions remains in *their* energy fields. This will inhibit the flow of their energies, increasing the likelihood of them feeling the void and preventing feelings of fulfillment. Although outwardly it may look as if they've gotten away with their actions, indirectly they're feeling the repercussions at the soul level.

It's especially difficult to forgive someone if we never see any outward signs of regret or remorse from them. This certainly stopped me from forgiving my mother when she was alive. In the years since her death, I've finally realized that she must have been abused as a child and she truly didn't know any better. She had her own unique journey on this earth, and since I had only partial insight into that, judging her, without all the facts, was taking up valuable space in my head. I finally realized it was in my best interest to let all that go, forgive her, clear my energy field, and move forward with my life.

For me personally, forgiving my mother was a long process. It happened in phases over time. What I've learned through the experience is that forgiveness is something that has to occur at both the mind and soul levels. I'd had several sessions with my counselor and thought I had forgiven my mother. Looking back now, I realize I had only forgiven her at the logical/mind level. At the soul level, I was still harboring feelings of resentment toward her.

It took two trips to Sedona to finally forgive my mother at all levels. Interpreting my dreams has led me to that conclusion. For most of my childhood and into early adulthood, whenever my mother turned up in my dreams, I was trying to punch her. After my first trip to Sedona, those dreams went away. In fact, I didn't dream about her at all. Once again, I thought I had finally forgiven her. However, it wasn't until after my last trip to Sedona that it became very clear that I had forgiven her, because she started appearing in my dreams again. However, instead of being the antagonist in my dreams, she has become just another player and is now at my side, supporting whatever I'm doing in the dream.

> Today I decided to forgive you. Not because you apologized, or because you acknowledged the pain that you caused me, but because my soul deserves peace.
>
> —Najwa Zebian

If you feel you need to forgive someone in order to move on with your life, it's important to seek out practitioners that can heal you at both the mind and soul level.

Self-Forgiveness

Sometimes anger and resentment are not aimed at others, but at ourselves. If we're harboring guilt and/or shame for our past transgressions, the best thing we can do is engage the right professionals/practitioners to help guide us through the process to forgive ourselves. Left untreated, these feelings will create emotional blockages and impair our connections to Home.

It took me a long time to grieve and process the loss of Devon and to understand that he'd had a manic episode, not a midlife crisis, and deal with the guilt of not being there for him. What I've since come to realize is that although the time he spent with me was some of the happiest of his life, I didn't (people need to find their own fulfillment) fill his void. If I had, he wouldn't have been motivated to change the medication which triggered his manic episode.

The fact that I wasn't there for his last eight months wouldn't have changed the outcome. He would have eventually taken his life. There was nothing more I could have done to save him, and when the universe offered an opportunity to spare myself from the pain of watching him slowly self-destruct, making the decision to go to Minnesota put me on my best path in life.

I've forgiven myself for not being there for Devon, and I now look at my time with Devon as a gift. Despite the tragic ending, for the first time in my life, I was in a relationship with a loving and supportive partner. Whenever there was conflict, we worked through our differences together and always managed to compromise. For someone who always ran from conflict and left things unresolved to fester, that was huge for me.

Conclusion

Leading a fulfilling life means staying connected, so we can receive the guidance that will help us make the right choices and keep us on the best paths in life. Staying connected to Home is synonymous with maintaining a healthy soul and a free-flowing energy field. This can be best achieved by:

- eliminating behaviors that lower our vibration,
- reducing circumstances that create interference,
- using our special skill/talent, to connect, as much as possible, and
- establishing a daily self-care regimen.

When self-care isn't enough, we need to engage experienced practitioners to help clear interference and emotional blockages in our energy fields (i.e., heal the connection to Home) and/or repair our fragmented souls (i.e., heal the soul).

Some day I hope to live in a world where family doctors will refer their patients to a professional that heals the soul, just as they would refer them to a cardiologist, counselor, or physiotherapist. I also hope that someday anyone who has received treatments for the soul will be able to file a claim against their health insurance. Until then, we need to practice self-care, pay attention to the signs of feeling the repercussions of emotional trauma and seek out experienced practitioners ourselves.

Section 3

It's Never Too Late to Take Care of Your Soul

If the concepts in this book are resonating with you, but you've been thinking that it's too late to start connecting and looking after your soul, this section will explain why it's never too late.

Reincarnation

When we die and our physical bodies cease to function, the piece of our soul that came here to earth releases its connection to the body, returns Home, and reintegrates back into the collective conscience. Then we make plans to come back here again. This cycle can repeat itself many times and is commonly referred to as *reincarnation*. Each lifetime we spend here on earth is called an *incarnation*.

I've read several theories on what happens after we leave here (earth) and before we come back again (from Home). Once again, I will condense into a couple of sentences what I've learned from several books. Although every book seems to have different details, they all seem to agree that once we arrive back Home, we assess our previous lifetimes and make plans to further our souls' growth by developing the objectives (or lessons we want to learn) for our next lifetime. How our next lifetime unfolds and whether we learn our lessons, is strongly influenced by the choices we make and the circumstances (family situation) under which we're born and raised.

In creating our objectives for our next lifetime, we also pick the people (souls) who will help teach us the lessons we need to learn. The most important of these people will be our parents. When sperm (from our biological fathers) penetrates the egg (from our biological mothers), it generates a chemical reaction and releases energy to create an ethereal (i.e., cannot be seen by the human eye) birth canal. It's through this canal that souls, coming back from Home, enter the earthly plane. It's also at that point in time when the mind, body and soul become one. If our vibrational levels were low when we left this earth, it is likely they will be low when our souls enter the birth canal. Our prior emotional blockages come along for the ride as well.

It's for this reason that it's never too late to start working on and healing our souls and raising our vibrations. We may not receive all the benefits in this lifetime, but we will certainly set ourselves up to be in better positions in our next lifetimes. Otherwise, if we continue engaging in low-level behaviors here on earth, it's likely we'll be surrounded by and attract low-level people and circumstances in our next lifetimes too. Although there are exceptions, in general, we can assume that the lower our vibrations, the less likely we're to connect, receive guidance, make the right decisions, and learn the lessons we set for ourselves, thus impacting fulfillment in this and future lifetimes.

If we don't learn our lessons, our souls don't develop while we're here on earth, and we keep coming back here with the same objectives. It can be a vicious cycle, and the lower our vibrations, the less likely we are to escape from it. One of the best ways to determine if you haven't learned your lessons over lifetimes is to see if you can recognize repeating patterns in your behaviors in this lifetime.

Repeating Patterns

The lessons we learn here on this earth foster the evolution of our souls and help differentiate us from the collective conscience. It's the primary reason we come here. Identifying repeating patterns in our behavior can be an indication we're not learning our lessons. Unfortunately, it can be difficult to identify repeating patterns because it requires a high level of self-awareness and deep introspection.

Repeated patterns of behavior typically manifest themselves as unhealthy coping mechanisms (e.g., drug abuse, hoarding, eating, shopping) used to escape emotional pain or fill the void. They tend to become addictions, be destructive, lower our vibrations, and cause pain and suffering for ourselves and the people around us. Depending on the situation, the time in between repeated behaviors can be short (in a matter of hours) or can be long and extend over days, weeks, months, or even years.

Ending the cycle means looking past the repeated behavior and understanding the root cause of the behavior. This can likely be accomplished through some form of rehab/counseling, which forces the individual to bring up and deal with emotional pain. Unfortunately, there is little incentive to do this because finding/

funding the right counseling resources can take time, while the emotional pain persists; whereas the repeated low-level behavior is typically cheaper, more attractive, more accessible and brings quick (albeit temporary) relief from the emotional pain.

The most obvious and common form of repeating pattern of low-level behavior is drug abuse. This is also the riskiest kind of repeating behavior because some drugs can be addictive. Not only are they repeating the behavior to dull the pain, but also because they're addicted to the drug. It's likely some of these people may have tried counseling and not been successful because they may not have received treatment at the soul level. Until soul treatments become part of our health and wellness systems, many of these cycles will continue.

Another common repeating pattern can be seen in people who jump from relationship to relationship, in an attempt to mask their emotional pain by filling the void with other people. They blame their partners for the issues in their relationships, and come to believe that, in changing partners, they'll improve their lives by finding someone better. Although not always the case, they eventually find themselves in similar situations with different people. Instead of looking inward and recognizing they're part of the problem in their relationships, they continue to look outward and blame others. I found myself in this pattern for many years.

From the time I had my first serious boyfriend at the age of fifteen until I was married at twenty-seven, I cycled through a number of guys. Looking back now, I realize that I toggled between the nice guys and the bad boys. It wasn't something I did consciously. Counseling has taught me that I was attracted to the bad boys because the drama that they brought into my life was very similar to the drama in my household growing up, and I was drawn to that type of relationship because it felt familiar to me. However, when the drama became too much, I'd break up with the bad boy to find a nice guy. Then I'd break up with the nice guy and look for a bad boy because I found the niceness boring and was craving the drama again.

There were ten years between my divorce and when I met Devon. During that time, I focused on how/why I was attracted to controlling and aggressive partners by reading self-help books and going to counseling. I desperately wanted to eliminate the repeating pattern. I'm not going to lie. It wasn't easy. There were a few "learning" relationships between my divorce and Devon. Although I found a couple of really nice men, I still hadn't done all the work I needed to be a good partner to them, and we broke up. I also endured one last very painful relationship with yet another narcissistic/manipulative man. It took far longer to end that relationship than I care to admit, but it was through that relationship that I finally broke the cycle and ended the repeating pattern.

When Devon came into my life, I had done the work on myself and was ready for a nice, loving, and supportive partner. Looking back, I believe in the time between my divorce and meeting Devon, I raised my vibration and was able to attract a higher-evolved soul, and I found myself in a loving mutually respectful, supportive relationship for the first time in my life.

One of the easiest things to do is to blame our repeating patterns on someone else and see ourselves as victims. In the end, if it's lowering our vibrations and impacting the quality of our lives, does it really matter whose fault it is? What's most important is looking past the blame and taking steps to end the repeating behaviors, raise our vibrations, and improve the quality of our lives, regardless of how we got there in the first place.

> If you focus on the hurt, you will continue to suffer.
> If you focus on the lesson, you will continue to grow.
>
> —Unknown

Every incarnation provides us with opportunities to end repeating patterns and learn new lessons, but if we continue to make bad choices in our lives, we can stay in the cycle over many lifetimes. The good news is that we've been provided with the means to escape from this cycle; we just have to listen and pay attention.

Imprinting

I struggled with the concept of reincarnation for a long time. It frustrated me because as we're born here on earth, our minds are wiped clean, and we forget everything we learned in our previous lifetimes. If we're expected to learn lessons and avoid repeating them over lifetimes, it would be helpful to leverage (in this lifetime) what we learned from past lifetimes. It was during the stream of consciousness I received after my last trip to Sedona that I understood that we do have the ability to pass information between lifetimes.

I will explain how this can happen, but first I want to demonstrate the concept by describing an episode of *Star Trek: The Next Generation*. I believe Gene Roddenberry (the creator of *Star Trek*) was clearly receiving messages and guidance from Home, and chose science fiction as his medium to communicate the messages.

This particular episode starts with the crew of the *Enterprise* encountering some form of turbulence, which affects the structural integrity of the ship. The situation degrades very quickly, and the entire ship blows up. Then we (the audience) are sent to commercial break, left to wonder what just happened. After the commercial break, we're even more perplexed, because we see the ship intact and the crew doing the same things they were doing at the beginning of the episode. Very quickly though, we see them back in the same situation; the ship encounters turbulence, blows up, and we go to commercial break again.

This pattern repeats itself several times throughout the episode. During each loop (i.e., incarnation), we see the crew make the same decisions, which leads them back to the incident where the ship explodes again. Eventually, through a number of loops, the crew begins to experience déjà vu, and they start realizing they're caught in a loop in time. However, each time they reach that conclusion, it's too late to change anything because the key decisions have already been made and the ship explodes again. Finally, they develop a way to pass information to themselves in the next loop. This leads them to make different decisions (in the final loop), and they're able to escape the turbulence, avoid the explosion and move on with their mission.

Our lifetimes are very similar. When we finally learn our lessons, such as when we end a repeating pattern and move on with our missions and continue our souls' growth, we leave an imprint on our soul. An imprint is wisdom that we carry across lifetimes and can be considered another form of guidance. It comes to us as a very strong sense of knowingness. It's knowledge/wisdom you have, but you can't explain how you've gained it. Like other forms of guidance, it helps shape your decisions and your path in life, but imprinting is a little different because you can access it when you're not connected (i.e., when you're experiencing interference or emotional blockages) to Home.

My daughter is what some people may refer to as an old soul. The wisdom she imparts has always been well beyond her years. Even as a small child, she would say some very profound things. I believe she is someone who has been here on earth many times, has learned many lessons (i.e., imprints) and is here to teach and guide others.

The most memorable time I believe I accessed my imprinting was when I was fourteen, in middle school, and had started hanging out with a new set of friends and engaging in low-level behaviors.

One Friday night, I was supposed to go to a party with a new friend. The plan was to get high (drugs and alcohol) and have sex with older boys. Shortly before I was to go to the party, I spoke with my new friend on the phone. I have a very clear memory of that phone conversation because my mother was hovering close by. As much as I wanted to rebel and go to that party, and knowing my actions would hurt and upset my mother, I also got a very strong sense (somehow I just knew) that in the long term I'd suffer more.

My desire to protect myself outweighed my desire to hurt my mother, and I decided not to go to the party, and more importantly, I decided to stop hanging out with my new friend that evening. Through the rest of middle school, my friend continued on a downward spiral.

By the time we started high school she had calmed down, found a really nice guy (who was a good friend of mine), and had settled into a great relationship with him. I got to know her all over again and remembered why I'd wanted to be her friend in middle school. Her laugh was infectious, and her smile could light up a room. I have many great memories of spending time with her in high school.

Although she didn't go to university with me, after we graduated from high school, we would often see each other on weekends. Unfortunately, the emotional pain from her past trauma caught up with her again, and she reverted back to her low-level coping behaviors. Eventually, the relationship that kept her stable for a number of years ended. In the meantime, I moved to another part of Canada, and we drifted apart.

Many years later, I was watching the national news on TV, and I saw her face posted next to a guy who was reported to be her boyfriend. They were both missing. It took another ten years before they found their bodies, side by side in a shallow grave. They had both been shot, execution style, in the back of the head. She and her boyfriend had ties to organized crime, and they had crossed the wrong people.

I often reflect back to that night in middle school, and I think about the choice I made. Long before I wrote this book, and long before my friend went missing, it has always stood out as one of the most critical choices in my life. I believe now it was imprinting and listening to the guidance from Home that led me to make the right decision that night.

I believe many people who use low-level or repeating behaviors to cope with anxiety, depression, and emotional pain from the past know the root causes of their pain, but they continue to mask it because it's easier than working through it. I know my friend knew the root cause of her low-level behaviors. It's a shame to waste a lifetime repeating unhealthy patterns, when there are healing techniques (albeit not well known) to break the cycle and improve the quality of this and other lifetimes.

In section 2, I discussed some powerful healing techniques. I will describe a few more techniques in this section to demonstrate that if you find the right professionals, you can cure emotional pain, eliminate low-level behaviors and move on with your missions in life.

Additional Soul-Healing Techniques

Logosynthesis

My counselor always told me that working through your issues was like peeling off the layers of an onion. Unfortunately, every time I thought I'd found the way to the core of my onion (i.e., I had worked through all my issues), I'd find another layer. I've finally come to realize that I may never get to the core of my onion, but I take comfort in knowing that my onion definitely has less layers than it once did.

By the time Devon entered my life, I had worked through a lot of my issues. When he and I met, I no longer craved the drama and dysfunction of my childhood. I was a fairly stable and calm person. However, under certain circumstances, I could quickly lose my calm and have an emotional outburst. During those outbursts, I'd completely lose control of my faculties and start screaming incoherently. Although these outbursts only happened once or twice a year, I was very ashamed of them, and I didn't want them to impact my relationship with Devon. So I decided to go see my counselor once again, peel off another layer of my onion, and work through (yet another) repeating behavior.

In the past, my counselor had success using a progressive healing technique called Logosynthesis, so he decided to use that technique for this issue as well. Logosynthesis leverages the power of well-formed sentences and thoughts (used to permeate an individual's energy field) as its primary mechanism for healing.

As always, we started the session with me closing my eyes and focusing inward. Then he asked me to repeat several sentences and phrases. Once I finished repeating the phrases, he asked for my impressions and feelings. Based on my responses, he formulated other sentences and words for me to repeat. After a few rounds of this, I could see the reason for these emotional outbursts was coming from my chest area, and in my mind's eye, I could see a black mass over my heart.

As I looked deeper into this black mass, I could see three little beings. Through discussions with these beings, I learned that as a young child I placed this black mass over my heart for protection. Whenever I was feeling extremely hurt, threatened, or panicked, these beings would trigger the emotional outburst. It had become their way of protecting me. As my counselor and I worked to remove them, they became more resistant and didn't want to leave. Over time, these beings had become sentient, and they feared that if they let go of me, they would cease to exist. It took a little time, but my counselor started negotiating with them and was finally able to convince them to leave. As part of the process, I thanked them for protecting me for so long, and I expressed that I didn't need the emotional outbursts anymore and that I was able to fend for myself now. Then I sent them on their way with love.

That was seven years ago. I've not had an emotional outburst since. Like the story of my trip into the blue light, I feared being judged, and I struggled with including the story in this book. However, the reason I included it and risked being judged, and the reason I felt compelled to tell the story, is the same reason I wanted to write this book. I want people to know there are techniques and things you can do to cure your emotional pain. Unfortunately, they haven't become mainstream yet, so you have to do the research and find the resources yourself. Most of all, though, you have to keep an open mind.

I find it astounding that my counselor was able to cure that repeating behavior in one session. I can't explain how or why that session unfolded the way it did. I remember during the session I wanted to stop, because even I thought it was absurd. However, I let go of my judgment and let it unfold as it did, and now, I'm grateful.

> The soul always knows what to do to heal itself. The challenge is to silence the mind.
>
> —Caroline Myss

Energy Healing

What I've only recently come to realize is that the treatments and methods I describe in this book (e.g., logosynthesis and soul retrieval) are all forms of energy healing. Energy healing (which can also be referred to as intuitive healing) is any type of method used to clear emotional blockages, raise our vibration and/or repair our connection to Home. I have received energy healing through sound, reiki, massage and guided meditation. I've also received energy healing in conjunction with traditional counseling. In general, it's been my experience that energy healing is more effective than traditional counseling.

Traditional counseling typically takes you through the front door (at a conscious level). If we're in denial of the root cause of our emotional pain, this method provides us with opportunities to lie to our counselors (and ourselves) about the true nature of our emotional pain and repeating patterns. Conversely, energy healing takes us through the back door (on a deeper subconscious level) and doesn't give us that opportunity to brush aside issues we don't want to face. The issues tend to bubble up out of nowhere and penetrate our consciousness. Before we know it, the issue is there in front of us. It's raw, it's exposed and we have no choice but to deal with it.

Denial is not the only reason some of us don't actively deal with our issues. Sometimes we've suppressed memories and emotions so deeply, our conscious minds can't retrieve them. I discovered some powerful repressed memories during a recent energy healing meditation. Within minutes of the start of the meditation a long-lost memory came through very clearly. I was in my childhood bedroom lying on my bed crying after receiving an undeserved punishment from my mother. Then I had a very clear vision of her entering my bedroom, berating me for crying and continuing with the punishment. It was in that moment (after 54 years) that I realized why I've suppressed emotion all my life. As a young child, I quickly learned if I expressed emotion, I would be punished for it.

Uncovering repressed memories and suppressed emotions means that sometimes energy healing sessions can be painful and produce a lot of tears, but in my experience it's been worth it. Because we're getting to the root cause quicker, energy healing tends to be faster and produce more permanent results. Having said that, there have been many times I've walked away from an energy healing session feeling like nothing happened because it's not always obvious. Such was the case after I cleared the three little beings from the front of my heart. It was over the course of the next year, as I noticed the subtle changes in my behaviour, that I realized the power in that one session.

I believe the reason energy healing is so effective is because in many cases it provides us with the means to process the pain and emotions, that we were ill equipped to deal with as they occurred. This particularly applies to those of us who have experienced trauma in childhood. The practitioner is there to facilitate and to encourage us to view the trauma with a mature adult lens and to help us file the emotions in the appropriate places in our minds, bodies and souls.

I can't believe how lucky (or perhaps it's another amazing coincidence) I was, that my counselor started using energy healing techniques while I was working with him. And it's not just counselors who are adapting energy healing as another skill/tool to help heal emotional trauma. Massage therapists, chiropractors, yoga and pilates instructors are learning energy healing techniques as well. This is because emotional blockages not only manifest in our minds as mental illness, but also in our bodies as physical ailments. The list of ailments is long, but auto-immune and gastro intestinal disorders are most common. If you have a chronic physical health issue, it's likely tied to an emotional blockage in your energy field.

I've focussed primarily on mental health issues because this book is really about connecting with the soul. That's the foundation for all energy healing, whether our blockages are physical or mental. Once we start energy healing, we will be intuitively guided to the places in our minds, bodies and souls that need healing. If we sense our unprocessed emotional issues have manifested more physically than mentally, we should seek out energy healing practitioners who also work on the body. Key words like "energy healing" or "intuitive healing" are good to use when looking for practitioners on the internet.

As with any profession, the strength and effectiveness of energy healing depends on the competency and skills of the practitioner. Effective energy healing is also greatly dependant on our commitment to the process. In making the most of energy healing, we should strive for the following:

- Engage multi-skilled practitioners,
- Keep an open mind (even when we think we're making it up),
- Be completely engaged (even when we think the process is ridiculous), and
- Recognize that although the healing process triggers more emotional pain, there is an end in sight (i.e., short term pain for long term gain).

Energy healing can be effective remotely (i.e., we don't need to be in the same location as our practitioners) but is most effective when we engage practitioners in places like Sedona, where the earth's energy vibrations are the highest.

Healing Past-Life Trauma

If you're having a hard time healing emotional issues in this lifetime, it's because they may be caused by trauma from a past life. This can explain why some people are more deeply affected by trauma than others. If an individual comes into this life with unhealed trauma from a past life, they may be more at risk of being affected by potentially traumatizing events in this life. Energy healing is the only way I know to heal past life trauma. Traditional counseling does not address it.

I recognize that believing in reincarnation is extremely difficult for some. Thankfully believing in past lives is not a prerequisite for receiving energy healing therapy. However, we will get more out of energy healing if we're open to the possibility of reincarnation. Remember, at one time in our history people undeniably thought the world was flat and those who initially thought otherwise, were mocked.

Karma

The simplest definition of the law of karma suggests that for every action there is an equal an opposite reaction. This implies that when we do something wrong to someone else, it comes back on us in some way. In fact, the negative actions, thoughts and emotions we direct toward someone else leaves deficits (sometimes referred to as "karmic debt") in our energy fields. These deficits act like magnets, and will beckon circumstances and experiences of a similar energy level, as payback for that situation.

In other words, everything you do to another, you inadvertently bring back on yourself. This applies to both good and bad karma. Many people think that paying it forward is a waste of time. However, if you perform an act of kindness, to someone who may never have an opportunity to do the same for you, the polarity of the little magnets in your energy field are reversed and, like bad karma, will attract positive experiences into your life. The problem with the law of karma is that payback can be quick and happen almost instantaneously, or very slow and happen over several years or even lifetimes.

Karma and Forgiveness - If after reading the piece on forgiveness in Section 2 you weren't persuaded to begin the forgiveness process, then perhaps understanding the relationship between karma and forgiveness, may help you to take that next step to heal your soul.

If someone has wronged us and we don't witness them receive some sort of payback in this lifetime, we may perceive life as not being fair and become even more bitter and resentful. These emotions, left to fester, can create interference and emotional blockages that will adversely impact the quality of our lives. The fact of the matter is, since we have no insight into the complexity and nature of another person's karmic debt, it's in our best interests to forgive that person and take the necessary steps to heal our soul, let go of the resentment from our energy fields and trust that the universe will eventually settle the other person's karmic debt. In other words, be safe in the knowledge that someday the law of karma will catch up to them (in this or a future lifetime), even if we never get to witness it.

Karma and Repeating Patterns – Once again, for the sake of brevity, I have provided a very simple definition of the law of karma. When in fact, karma and how we create our karmic debt, is quite complex. This is because our karmic debt is not just tied to our transgressions, but it is also tightly tied to our life's lessons and repeating patterns. As we end repeating patterns, learn our lessons and leave imprints on our soul, not only do we clear emotional blockages and interference, we are also quite likely clearing karmic debt and setting ourselves up for getting back on our best path in this and future lives.

Conclusion

Reincarnation gives us that opportunity for a do-over, which means it's never too late to start looking after our souls, raising our vibrations to help us receive guidance, and accessing our imprinting to find fulfillment in this lifetime and lifetimes to come.

Energy healing provides us with a means to uncover repressed memories and suppressed emotions, process emotional pain from past (and past life) trauma and heal the connection to our soul. Staying committed to the process and finding practitioners who use energy healing in conjunction with other healing treatments such as massage therapy, yoga, chiropractic care and counseling is a very effective means to eliminate repeating patterns of behavior and cure certain types of chronic physical and mental health issues.

Identifying repeating patterns of behavior, understanding the root causes of our low-level behaviors and seeking treatments to eliminate them, will help clear our karmic debt and leave imprints on our souls that can be accessed over lifetimes. This can be achieved through self-awareness, deep introspection and learning to take responsibility for our actions.

The ultimate excuse for making bad decisions and repeating low-level behaviors is to blame our parents and our upbringing and to think of ourselves as victims. That was certainly my early thought patterns. However, in one of his books, Wayne Dyer taught me that we can only blame our demise on our parents (or lack thereof) for so long. At some point in our lives, we became adults responsible for own decisions and choices, and it's at that point that we need to accept accountability for the states of our lives.

Many of the great thinkers and spiritual leaders of today (Oprah comes to mind first) started life in less-than-ideal circumstances. However, at some point (likely by accessing her imprinting), she started making decisions that led her to the great success she has achieved today. As a society, we tend to believe Oprah found success because she is "special," when in fact, there are countless "ordinary" people who didn't achieve Oprah's level of fame but took charge of their lives, found fulfillment, and put themselves on a better path. Since they're not famous, we just don't hear their stories.

> I am not a product of my circumstances. I am a product of my decisions.
>
> —Stephen Covey

Being successful and finding fulfillment in life isn't something that can only be experienced by the privileged or "special" people. In fact, viewing someone like Oprah as being privileged and special is just another tactic generated by our egos to provide us with another excuse for not taking charge of our own lives (i.e., taking risks), and prevents us from believing that we, too, have the power to turn our lives around. That power can help us break the cycle of lifetimes and get our souls on the path to recovery. The choice is ours, and it's never too late.

Section 4

Thinking at the Soul Level

Ending repeating patterns isn't the only means by which we can learn lessons, imprint, and foster our souls' growth here on earth. We also have opportunities to learn lessons by finding healthier means (than low-level repeating behaviors) to cope with traumatizing events. It's during difficult times that we have the option to turn to low-level behaviors to cope, or to choose healthier coping mechanisms. One of the best healthy coping strategies I've found is learning to think about life at the soul level.

Thinking at the soul level means being able to stand back (almost like an objective bystander) and look at your life through the lens of your untarnished soul. It means removing the judgment and bias created by your ego and looking at your life as if you were still at Home, viewing yourself here on earth.

Learning to think at the soul level is a progression that happened for me in two stages:

The first stage (soul level I) of thinking at the soul level allows us to not only recognize repeating patterns, but also to see beyond the painful and traumatizing experiences in our lives, view them as "blessings in disguise" or "silver linings," and even progress to the point where we're grateful for the painful experience. Thinking this way also provides us with an opportunity to imprint and carry the wisdom gained into our next lifetimes. Being able to look back and consistently derive the positive from bad situations is a good indicator that we have learned to think at soul level I.

Thinking at soul level II means that we're not just able to look back and be grateful for a painful experience. Thinking at soul level II challenges us to be grateful while we're experiencing the pain. In thinking at soul level II, we're mindful that part of our purposes here on earth is to grow, and without the painful experience, we may not achieve our objectives for this lifetime.

To use an analogy, the difference between thinking at level I and level II is the difference between how a swimmer and a surfer deal with turbulent waves in the ocean. A swimmer is actually in the water and will get tossed around, even getting pulled down under if the water is really rough. A swimmer may also become disoriented and lose sight of the beach (his final destination). Conversely, a surfer rides on top of the waves, is somewhat buffered from the turbulence in the water, and can usually see the beach. He can still experience some ups and downs and can fall off the board, but he can use the board to catch the next big wave and get back on top of the water again.

In this scenario, the surfer has the advantage because he isn't as affected by the water (the emotions). Riding on top of the waves, he sees the destination and can actually carve the best path forward, whereas the swimmer is at the complete mercy of the waves (i.e., feels the full intensity of the emotions) and can even lose sight of the destination. Once the swimmer reaches the beach, he can look back and see what he did wrong (level I), but the surfboard (level II) buffered the surfer from experiencing the waves and allowed him to get to the beach sooner. In life, we must strive to be surfers and use our soul-level thinking as our surfboard and our primary coping mechanism.

Thinking at Soul Level I—Blessings in Disguise

I believe my greatest achievement in life has been, that I broke the cycle of abuse in my family. I didn't abuse my daughter. Although I was far from the perfect parent, once the divorce was finalized, I did my best to raise my daughter in a very loving and supportive environment. She won't have to deal with the legacy of generations of abusers (I can only assume my mother was abused as well), and she won't pass that on to her children in this world. At twenty-one, my daughter is already attracting higher vibrating souls than I did at her age. I believe, through her, I've improved the lineage of this family here on earth.

When I look back on my life, there are two reasons why I believe I was able to break the cycle of abuse:

The first reason is that I received a higher education and learned that abuse is socially and morally unacceptable and (in extreme cases) illegal. It's ironic that my mother was the one who encouraged me to go to university. She really didn't have an opportunity to receive an education beyond her high school diploma. She married and had children when she was very young. Although she took occasional jobs as a bookkeeper, for the most part, she was a stay-at-home mom. Despite that, she recognized the value in higher education. She knew I was smart and would have no problem earning a degree. For as long as I can remember, she told me I was going to university and that I didn't have a choice. For that, I will be forever grateful.

The second reason I broke the cycle of abuse is that I learned alternative means to disciplining children besides berating and beating them. There is no doubt in my mind that the abuse I received from my mother was meant to be discipline (i.e., just a spanking) for what she perceived as bad behavior on my part. The problem with this type of discipline is that it can escalate out of control, and my mother's response was usually grossly disproportionate to my behavior. What she intended to be a spanking, quickly turned into a beating that was accompanied by an onslaught of verbal and emotional degradation. In other words, discipline quickly turned to abuse. Learning there were alternatives to discipline, that didn't involve spanking, was a game changer for me.

My ex-husband had a degree in psychology and taught me that positive reinforcement (instead of discipline) is a much more powerful way to mold a child's behavior. Negative reinforcement (i.e., abuse) just tends to make children feel bad about themselves, whereas positive reinforcement (praising, rewarding a child's good behavior and ignoring their bad behavior) builds self-esteem. Not surprisingly, positive reinforcement promotes the flow of positive energy, while negative reinforcement creates noise and interference. I will always be grateful that my ex-husband showed me a better path forward, and sad that we were not able to take that path together.

Thinking at soul level I, I've been able to look past the resentment and the anger to recognize that the two people who disappointed me the most in this life were also two of my biggest teachers. They helped me grow as a human being, learn my lessons here on earth, and further develop my soul.

I could have chosen the easy way, thought of myself as a victim and revictimized my daughter. I could have chosen not to change my ways and mirror my mother's ways. Instead, I chose to use alternative means to discipline and raise her, to look at the situation through the lens of my soul and to see the silver linings. This is why I think of myself as a survivor and someone who has not only learned from the pain of my past, but who has thrived because of it.

> It's nice to look back at your life and see things as lessons, not regrets.
>
> —Rihanna

Thinking at Soul Level II—Painful Endings Are New Beginnings

In most cases, after we endure trauma, our lives change dramatically, and we start experiencing what is sometimes called the "painful ending." The life we once lived ceases to exist, and we have to carve a new path for ourselves. The first time I experienced a painful ending was after my divorce and my mother's death. Those early years after the divorce were difficult. But making new friends, reading self-help books and developing on a spiritual level defined my "new beginning" and helped me find fulfillment. It was during that time that I started my own business and learned about many of the concepts I describe in this book. I didn't know it at the time, but I was learning to think at soul level I. Then I met Devon and started experiencing my first truly supportive partner. Life was good for a number of years. Then, very quickly, in the span of about six weeks, it all changed, and my second painful ending began.

The first blow was when my daughter left home to go to university. Being a single mom, I felt the effects of an empty nest more than most. The second blow was when Devon broke up with me, and the third blow was when he took his own life. Dealing with all that loss in my life was overwhelming. Despite all the pain, I was able to realize that I had been through something similar, and for the second time in my life, I was experiencing another painful ending. During my lowest times, I was able to find comfort in knowing there would be another "new beginning" on the horizon. Knowing that I survived and thrived after the last painful ending gave me faith that eventually this situation would turn around too. This is thinking at soul level II.

As I write this book, my new beginning is still shaping. I don't know what the future has in store for me, but I'm excited for it. I still have times when I lament the past and wish Devon was still here. But I realize that I can't change what happened, and I must accept it. Thinking at soul level II, I understand that there is purpose to the pain. I truly believe I chose this path before I came here. Understanding the detrimental affect this experience had on my soul and taking the steps to heal it properly, has not only helped my soul further evolve, but has also deepened my human experience. Capturing it in a book has been one of the most rewarding things I've ever achieved. It's my hope that this book will influence others to think at the soul level as well.

Mastering Soul-Level Thinking—Shaping your New Beginning

When we're able to look back, deduce the lessons learned, and see the good from past painful experiences, it becomes easier to cope with challenging times as we adjust and accept the changes that come along with our new beginning. However, the uncertainty that comes along with change can add to the stress we may already be experiencing. Instead of sinking further into despair, mastering soul-level thinking teaches us this is an opportunity and the perfect time to shape our new lives. It's the perfect time to set intentions, use the law of attraction, and provide the universe with a vision of our new lives.

Setting Intentions

In section 2, I described intentions as one of the more powerful forms of thought. So it's important to know that how we construct our intentions has a direct impact on how effective they are. We don't want our intentions to prescribe how our future comes together; instead, we want to leave them open ended and focus on the end result. This is because we want to give the universe the space it needs to rally around us and provide the support (i.e., people, information, money) that it needs to create our future in ways we could not imagine.

Some people set intentions by creating vision boards (using pictures). Others just write them on a piece of paper or in a journal. I've used and have had success with all these techniques. Intentions should be worded positively (i.e., no negative language), use active language, and have a directive tone.

After my divorce, and before I started reading self-help books in earnest, I didn't understand I was going through a new beginning. Once I moved into the new house and began deepening my spiritual beliefs, I spent time trying to make sense of the divorce and everything else that had happened. That's also when I started learning about setting intentions and the law of attraction. Since my daughter was struggling (she was also feeling the impact of the divorce) at that time, I decided to put her needs ahead of everything, even my career. The intention I set at that time, was that I wanted more flexibility (to be able to leave work and pick her up from school), to work less (take more vacation), and to make more money.

Once we plant intentions, it's time to let go and let the universe work its magic. It can be difficult to move on though, because as humans, we inherently like to maintain control, and our egos have a hard time letting go.

Letting Go

Sometimes in life, when things just don't appear to be going our way, we hang on tightly and try to control the situation. We resist change and try to keep things the way they are. When we're controlling a situation, the energy around the situation becomes restricted. This hinders the free flow of energy and prevents the universe from organizing around and resolving the matter to the best outcome and the highest good of all involved.

Conversely, when we want a situation to change, we try to control the outcome and force things to happen in certain ways. This can involve manipulating and bullying others to get what we want. These are low-level behaviors that create interference and restrict the flow of energy around ourselves and the situation. We may achieve the outcome we wanted, but it may have been a result of choices/actions that generated bad karma and placed us on a less-than-optimal path in life.

Mastering soul-level thinking means we have to believe that the universe will organize and make it happen in the best way possible. This is why setting the proper intention is so important. Instead of trying to control the situation, think about what you want in life and then set your intention and let the universe deliver results in the most unexpected and wonderful ways.

Although the intention I set didn't prescribe "how" it was to happen, I felt the only way I could possibly achieve that outcome was to continue being a consultant, but be self-employed. Although all the books I'd read told me to let go and leave it up to the universe, I found it impossible. I wanted everything to change, and I wanted it to change *then*.

Instead of letting the universe do its thing, I intervened and started knocking on doors and looking for opportunities to leave my employer and find self-employment. I had to be careful though, because there was a noncompete clause in my employment contract. This meant it was illegal for me to work directly for any of my employer's existing clients. It was during this time that one of my employer's clients made an offer to hire me as an independent consultant. Accepting this offer meant I'd breach the noncompete clause.

I talked to two other consultants and a lawyer about making this move. They all said that the likelihood of being prosecuted for breaching my noncompete clause was low, because my employer couldn't keep me from making a living. For that reason, most companies rarely enforce their noncompete clauses.

After a lot of thought, I decided that leaving my employer for an existing client would be bad karma. I live and work in a small city, and I thought it would be too much of a risk to burn that bridge. That's when I finally decided to let go. Although I wasn't enjoying my job and I was worried about my daughter, I let it all go.

Waiting for the Universe to Work Its Magic

While we're waiting for the universe to work its magic, interference and emotional blockages can slow the process and even prevent it from happening. This is why we need to feed our souls and do our best to focus on and keep the energy around us clean and free flowing. During the waiting period, we need to do our best to live in the moment and show gratitude for the parts of our life that are good, and we need to keep the faith that the universe will provide for us. The problem is the universe can create things instantaneously, or it can take months. Along with keeping our energy field clean and demonstrating patience, we need to start paying attention for coincidences and other signs of synchronicity. Waiting is difficult, but it can also be rewarding.

While I waited for the universe to create my future, I journaled coincidences, kept reading books, and continued my spiritual development.

> Patience is not the ability to wait, but how you act while you're waiting.
>
> —Joyce Meyer

Divine Timing and Synchronicity

After we've set our intentions and while we're keeping our energy fields clean, we have to be patient because results can take longer than expected. Mastering soul-level thinking means understanding that there is such a thing as "divine timing," and we may have to wait for circumstances to line up like dominos. You'll know when things are starting to fall into place, because you'll start receiving signs/guidance messages (usually in the form of coincidences and synchronicity) to direct your life down a certain path.

After I decided to let go, it took three months, but I finally got a call from a colleague who needed someone with my skills. There was synchronicity in that call, because this colleague was one of the last people I'd spoke to, before I made my final decision to let go. Although the intent of that prior conversation was to ask for her opinion on breaching my noncompete clause with my employer, through that conversation, I unintentionally planted a seed. A few months later, when an opportunity crossed her desk, the seed sprouted, and she thought of me. Once I signed the contract, quit my job, and started my own consulting company, synchronicity and coincidences happened that placed people in my path just as I needed them.

Setting up my own company was easy (a sign I was on the right path), and I worked on that first contract for a year. Although working on my first project as an independent consultant was very challenging, the work experience was invaluable. It gave me confidence I didn't have, provided me with opportunities to build an extensive network (it was a large project) of like-minded individuals, and set me up for future successes. If I had taken the earlier opportunity with my existing client (the less optimal path), I definitely wouldn't have gained that work experience and may not have achieved the same level of success in my business. In this way, I'm convinced the universe created a better outcome for me than the job I tried to find for myself.

Once I finished that project, I easily found work at another company. This was when my full intentions were realized. That new client allowed me to work from home, and I was able to pick my daughter up at school every day. I raised my rates and was making more money than when I'd worked for my former employer. This afforded me the luxury of taking more time off. I've worked steadily over the last fifteen years and always found clients that let me work from home or leave work early.

When we let go and let the universe sort things out for us, we usually end up with a situation far better than what we could have created for ourselves. Mastering soul-level thinking is having complete faith and trust in the universe. It also means letting go of fear and doubt.

Managing Fear and Doubt

Fear and doubt will cause you to hang on tight to a situation and lose faith in the universe. These emotions create interference and lower your vibration. After you've set intentions (at a time when you should be focusing on feeding your soul and keeping your energy field clear), your ego (as mine did) will step into high gear and plant thoughts in your head to be impatient, lose faith in the universe, and try to control the situation. When we master soul-level thinking, we're able to identify the thoughts that are being driven by our egos and replace them with thoughts to keep our energy fields clear and support the universe for our highest good.

Minimizing fear and doubt provides the space for us to focus on recognizing and interpreting guidance from Home. As it's the strength of the guidance, that will give us the courage to act. Then, when we do act, we typically need to be prepared to take a risk.

Taking (Calculated) Risks

When we're making big changes in our lives, we will more than likely be taking financial (potential to lose money) or emotional (lose support of loved ones) risks. Fear and doubt will drive thoughts that will keep us from taking these risks. There will be constant chatter inside our heads as the needs of our souls conflict with the needs of our egos.

No matter how much I feel making a certain decision and taking a new path is right for me, I won't move forward without first calculating the risks. Taking calculated risks helps the ego let go and reduces the amount of conflict and chatter in your head. Before I decide to take a risk, I always assess whether I have a safety net or a backup plan. For example, when I left full-time employment and started my own business, I was quite certain I could get my old job back, if I failed. By not breaching my non-compete clause, I created that safety net, because I left that business relationship in very good standing.

Having said that, there have been times when I've taken a leap of faith without a backup plan because the guidance from Home has been so strong. Taking risks is a balancing act. For the most part, I always try to let common sense prevail.

Aside from starting my own business, another big risk I took in my life was taking time off work (i.e., walking away from my clients and my existing contracts) to heal the emotional blockages created by not dealing with the breakup with Devon and his death.

I had some savings and considered that to be my safety net. However, I didn't know how long I'd need to heal, and there was no way of knowing if I'd find work again. I took five months off work and spent three months traveling. I stayed in contact with my clients during that time. Although my soul healed in those five months and I was ready to return to work, once I returned home, I received very strong guidance to start writing this book.

Prior to arriving home, I had done some research about book writing and learned that most people need dedicated and uninterrupted time to write a book. I was certain I couldn't write a book and work full time. By this time, my savings had run out, and I was worried about money. Although I had a small amount of work from one of my long-standing clients, my ego was pushing me to search for full-time work. Since the guidance to write this book was very strong, it gave me the confidence to graciously accept the part-time work, ignore my ego's desire to find full-time work, and start writing this book in earnest.

At times fear and doubt crept in, made me lose faith, and pushed me off my surfboard into the emotional waters. However, over time, it became very apparent to me that the universe supported me through this whole initiative. On those days, when my panic over where the next dollar was coming from was highest, I'd get unsolicited out-of-the-blue offers for small amounts of work. I accepted the part-time work and was able to keep writing and quell my ego's fear of financial ruin.

Then, as I was finishing up the first complete rough draft of my book, I got an offer for a fifteen-month contract. I returned to work full-time and was able to finish/refine the book over weekends and holidays. Having that fifteen-month contract has provided me with the financial stability I need while I wait for the universe to shape my new beginning and the next phase of my life. It's interesting and coincidental that the very topics I was writing about unfolded like a play in front of me.

Once again, taking a risk paid off. I was able to take the time to heal my soul and write this book, without going deeply into debt or bankruptcy.

Leveraging the Law of Attraction at Any Time

The last section—"Mastering Soul-Level Thinking—Shaping Your New Beginning"—was really a crash course in the law of attraction. Although that section describes using the law of attraction for shaping new beginnings, the law of attraction can be used to improve your life at any time. I've used the law of attraction many times in my life, and even when I didn't know I was using it. I believe my vision of raising my daughter on a quiet, family-oriented cul-de-sac (prior to my divorce) was so strong that it became an intention, even though it was never committed to paper. In fact, if one were to do the research, I bet we would discover many instances of people using the law of attraction without even knowing it.

The most memorable time I used it was when I purchased a cottage on the ocean.

I live in Nova Scotia, a province in Canada that's almost entirely surrounded by the Atlantic Ocean. I love the ocean because it makes me feel better when I'm looking at it, swimming in it, and just generally being around it. After I started my business and things were going well, I decided I wanted a cottage on the ocean. I did the math and realized that even though my business was thriving, I didn't have the money to buy the cottage. So I decided to test the law of attraction (I had absolutely nothing to lose), and I set my intentions for purchasing a small cottage on the ocean. I placed a picture of the type that I liked and made a small vision board in my journal. Then I let go, and quite frankly, I literally forgot about it, as I became very busy with work and single parenting. The months passed.

During that time, my beloved aunt passed away and left me a small sum of money. Not wanting to waste her hard-earned money, I placed it in savings and carried on with life. Then one weekend, I went away to visit friends at their cottage on a lake. As I sat on their deck, I looked out over the lake and once again thought about having my own cottage on the ocean. I quickly came to the conclusion that there was no way I could maintain another property (in addition to my house) on my own. I decided that what I really needed was a cottage that was also a condominium.

Then I started thinking about the ideal place where I'd like to have my cottage/condo, and I thought of a place called Hubbards. Hubbards is a quaint little rural community in Nova Scotia. Sitting on my friend's deck that morning I said to myself, "Too bad I couldn't find a condo in Hubbards." I chuckled to myself, because I had never heard of condos in rural Nova Scotia before.

Later that day, as I was driving on the highway back home, it started raining quite heavily. I decided to take the next exit off the highway and take a longer, slower route home. It just so happened the next exit would take me directly through Hubbards. As I turned left to take the alternate route off the highway, I saw a sign that said "Condos for Sale." I couldn't believe my eyes! I committed the phone number to memory and called as soon as I got home.

I purchased a beautiful cottage/condo directly on the ocean in Hubbards. The cottage was part of a well established rental property. There was staff in place, and I already had bookings the day I purchased it. Because it was an income property, I could afford to purchase it, and I used the money my aunt left me for the down payment.

We used the cottage whenever it wasn't rented, and it became my happy place. Once again, the universe provided what I asked for, in a way that I never thought possible.

The uncanny thing about this story is that I'd truly forgotten about the little vision board I'd placed in my journal. As I prepared to write this book, I reread all my old journals and was shocked when I saw the picture (of my future cottage) I'd placed in my journal and how similar it was to the cottage/condo that I eventually purchased. It was truly a miracle.

> You get in life what you have the courage to ask for.
> —Oprah Winfrey

The Law of Attraction and Cocreating

When your energy field is clear of blockages and free flowing, the universe can rally around you and provide you with the life you imagine. This is also how the law of attraction works best for you.

If you're interested in knowing more about the law of attraction (or the Secret), there are many books dedicated to the topic. I only mention it in this book because there is overlap between maintaining a healthy soul and activities required to be successful using the law of attraction.

Many people use the law of attraction to create abundance in their lives. However, that can be dangerous because creating abundance alone doesn't necessarily mean you'll find fulfillment. The law of attraction works best when you set intentions that are based on guidance you receive from Home. This is called *cocreating* and will lead you to a life beyond just abundance and into fulfillment.

The Journey to Fulfillment

Finding fulfillment is a journey, not a destination. So it's important to note that once we do the work to heal from emotional trauma, we may not feel fulfilled. That's because even though we've eliminated/reduced our emotional pain, we could still be feeling the void. Remember: the void is created because our connection wasn't clear, we couldn't receive/listen to the guidance from our souls, and we were not on our best paths in life. In other words, clearing emotional blockages alone may not eliminate feelings generated by the void.

Thankfully, clearing emotional blockages brings clarity and places us in better positions to receive guidance. Then it's up to us to set our intentions, use the law of attraction, and work with the universe to cocreate our best paths in life. While we wait for the universe to work its magic, we need to keep our energy fields clear, practice self-care, look for signs of and act on synchronicity and work on elevating our thinking to the soul level. It's during this time we'll find pockets of fulfillment. Focus on the pockets because gradually they'll grow, and feelings of fulfillment will reduce and eventually even eliminate the void.

Enlightenment

In Section 1 of this book I indicate that our soul's come here (earth) because they want to experience life on a different level. They want to feel what it's like to breathe air and to experience what it's like to taste, touch, feel (other emotions besides love), hear, and see. Which is true, but I believe our ultimate purpose for coming here is to attain *enlightenment*. I expect there are many different definitions for what it means to be enlightened. I believe it means to elevate our vibrations to the same frequency as Home, while we're here on earth.

This became very clear to me during a recent meditation as these words came through:

> It's not about loving others. It's not about being loved.
> It's about being love.
> —Margaret-Ann Hall

Since the essence of the energy at Home is love, I interpreted these words to be about enlightenment. I also think it means that the more that we practice "being love" and "loving others", "being loved" will happen naturally. I searched for this quote (and ones similar) on the internet. I couldn't find another quote like it. For that reason, I've decided to claim it as my own.

I don't think I've come close to enlightenment yet, but I now believe it's attainable. Although I don't expect to achieve it in this lifetime or even the next few after that, I feel like I may have started a good foundation. As I tell my clients when I'm helping them implement IT solutions, "Baby steps. We've got to start somewhere".

Conclusion

I use the term *soul-level thinking* in this book to describe how my thinking has taken on a soul-based perspective. Seeing the positive outcomes and lessons learned after we have recovered from our painful experiences, means we've learned to think at soul level I. Understanding that good will come from them and that there is purpose while we're still enduring the fallout from painful experiences, means we've learned to think at soul level II. Mastering soul-level thinking means we understand that the emotional pain is an ending and that we have the power to shape our new beginning.

For the skeptical reader, it's easy to read this book and discount the experiences and concepts that I describe. I completely understand because I've discounted them many times myself. However, the more things happened to me, the more I had to search for answers. This book is how I've sewn it all together, to make sense of how my life has unfolded.

I don't think I'm alone in adapting a soul-based perspective on life. As I looked for quotes to include in this book, it became apparent to me that others have adapted a similar perspective. It was most obvious in these two quotes from Steve Jobs (the founder of Apple):

> Follow your heart and intuition. They somehow already
> know what you truly want to become.

You can't connect the dots moving forward; you can only connect them looking backwards. So you have to trust the dots will connect somehow in your future. You have to trust in something—your gut, destiny, life, karma, whatever. This approach has never let me down, and it has made all the difference in my life.

I don't have insight into his entire belief system, but clearly he believed in some of the basic principles described in this book. I'm hoping this book causes you to pause for a moment and consider the possibility of living life through the lens of your own beautiful soul.

Epilogue

When I look back on the last fifty-four years, I believe the experiences that have impacted me the most were my trip into the blue light and the stream of consciousness I received to write this book. I will share one more experience that helped restore my faith and bring me hope during one of the most trying times in my life.

Devon was agnostic and didn't believe in life after death or anything that he couldn't see or touch. During our time together, we had some healthy debates about the differences in our belief systems. When these discussions were over, we would always agree to disagree, and I'd always say to him, "If you go first, you have to come back and communicate with me."

About three or four days after he passed, I was alone at home when I heard a commotion on my deck. When I went outside, I saw a bird fluttering around and noticed it had a broken wing. I recruited my daughter and her friend to help me capture it and bring it to the nearest wildlife sanctuary. Through the whole experience, I had a feeling it was a visit from Devon. I felt it was his way of letting me save him, because I wasn't able to save him while he was here.

After that encounter, I started seeing white feathers around our house and felt they were his way of communicating and saying hi to me. However, since we have a number of throw cushions that shed white feathers, I once again discounted the experience and told myself I was reading too much into the situation. Although white feathers still appeared, I decided to ignore them.

As the one-year anniversary of his death approached, I began to feel very anxious. I hadn't spoken to any of his family or friends in a year, and I wanted to reach out to his oldest son to see how he was doing. However, I was worried that contact from me might increase any stress that he may be feeling. I resisted the urge to contact him and suffered in silence. Two days before the anniversary of his death, Devon's ex-wife contacted me and encouraged me to reach out to his oldest son.

He was out of town visiting family at the time, so I texted him, told him I was struggling, and asked him how he was doing. Since Devon had raised him to be agnostic, I felt as though I had to be very cautious and choose my words carefully. If Devon was communicating with me, it was likely he was communicating with his son too. I very carefully mentioned that since his Dad had a larger-than-life presence here on earth, it would make sense that he'd make himself known from the other side. If he felt his Dad around him, it likely wasn't his imagination.

Even with everything that I've experienced, I was still shocked when he replied and told me that he felt his father was communicating and asked me to keep an eye out for white feathers for him. Until that moment, I had not told anyone about the significance of white feathers since Devon had passed away.

After we concluded our conversation, it was time to take the dog out to do her business. As I rounded the corner to go to her usual spot in the back of our home, several birds that were on the ground took flight into the trees. Except for one. One bird stayed on the ground, and as the dog and I progressed down the path, the bird started bouncing (six to eight inches in the air) across our path about ten to twenty feet in front of us. It looked to me as if the bird was jumping for joy. Once again, I felt this was a visit from Devon and he was expressing his delight in the conversation I just had with his son.

Once the bird crossed our path, it stopped bouncing, but it continued walking on the ground and kept looking back at us. In my mind, I said, "Devon, if that's you, make the bird do something." I fully expected the bird to take flight. Instead, it immediately stopped and pooped in its tracks. Devon had a great sense of humour in life; it appears he kept it on the other side too.

Since that time, my daughter and I often see white feathers around our home. Because we have cushions that shed white feathers, we don't interpret every feather as a message from Devon. The feathers we notice the most are the ones that show up in the strangest of places, where they hadn't been two seconds before, and just at the right time (when we need encouragement the most).

If nothing else, I hope this last story and the rest of this book conveys the message that there is more to this existence than we can see, feel, and touch. I hope it inspires you to pay attention to that next coincidence or reconsider some of your own past experiences. Most of all, I hope it encourages those of you who may be struggling and looking for a better path forward, to take that next terrifying step.

You're not alone. The universe will always be there to support you. You just have to take care of your soul and believe.

The Universe is always speaking to us. Sending us little messages, causing coincidences and serendipities, reminding us to stop, to look around, to believe in something else, something more.

—Nancy Thayer

Acknowledgments

I'd like to thank the following people who have been on this journey with me:

To my daughter Daphne-Jean "DJ", for being the light of my life and wise beyond your years. Being your mother has been my greatest pleasure in life. I love you more than you could ever imagine.

To my father Fred Hall, for instilling such a strong work ethic, igniting my passion for technology and doing your best to be there for me. To his partner, Rose, for taking care of my father, for letting us invade your home and taking on the role of grandmother to my daughter.

To my sister Laury Hall and her partner Trevor, for letting me stay with you on my healing journey and being there when I needed you most.

To my dear friend Margaret Sterns for always being in my court, for sharing your experiences as a mom, for supporting my business and being the most positive female role model in my life. In striving to be more like you, I became a better person. Most of all, because you believed in me, I started believing in myself.

To my family from Kaytyon Court, Tammy, Ed, Sheila, Kevin, Debbie, Mark, Tracy, Terry, Asa, Eggert and all their children. Thanks for all the laughter, always having my back and being the best neighbors I could have ever hoped for.

To my surrogate children Sophia, Colton, George, and Dallas. It has been an absolute pleasure watching you grow and become adults. I love you to the moon and back.

To my friend Graham Patterson, for being such an amazing role model and inspiring me to believe in myself. It's been twenty years, and you're still the best consultant I've ever worked with. Thanks for being the big brother I never had, for introducing me to your wife, Brenda (another incredible female role model), and for inviting me on your adventures.

To my friends the Maxwells, Mike and Cindy, for supporting my business, for always letting me overstay my welcome and for taking care of me during a time when my soul needed it most.

To my doctor, Diane D'Arcy, for caring about me and my daughter, coaching me during the infant stage, and being another positive female role model.

To my counselor, Phillippe Islor, for helping me find myself. I wouldn't be the person I am today without you. From the bottom of my heart, thank you.

To my Angel Therapy Practitioner, Karen Forrest, for receiving messages on my behalf, for coaching me on recognizing guidance and giving me the confidence to interpret it myself.

To my friend Kevin MacDonell, for coming into my life at just the right time and providing such valuable feedback on my manuscript.

To all the practitioners at Spirt Quest in Sedona, for helping heal my soul and providing me with some of the last nuggets I needed to finish this book.

To my friends in Minnesota, Paula Rivet and Jean Esslinger, for helping make my time in Minneapolis, the best it could have been.

To my dearly departed friends who left this world too soon. Kim Lockyer, I will never forget you. Carol Lemire, I still miss you, and I know you would have enjoyed this book.